Journey
OF THE
Heart

OTHER BOOKS BY JOHN WELWOOD

Journey
OF THE
Heart

THE PATH OF
CONSCIOUS
LOVE

John Welwood, Ph.D.

HarperPerennial
A Division of HarperCollinsPublishers

Grateful acknowledgment is made to the following for permission to reprint portions of copyrighted material:

Robert Bly:
For his translation of Goethe's "The Holy Longing." From *News of the Universe: Poems of Twofold Consciousness*, by Robert Bly. Copyright 1984 by Robert Bly.

Random House, Inc.:
From *Nature, Man, and Woman*, by Alan W. Watts. Copyright 1958 by Pantheon Books, Inc. Reprinted by permission of Pantheon Books, a Division of Random House, Inc.

From *The Work of Craft*, by Carla Needleman. Copyright 1979 by Carla Needleman. Published by Alfred A. Knopf, Inc.

Viking Penguin Inc., a division of Penguin Books USA, Inc.:
From *The Rainbow* by D.H. Lawrence. Copyright 1943 by Frieda Lawrence.

From "New Heaven and New Earth," in *The Complete Poems of D. H. Lawrence*, collected and edited by Vivian de Sola Pinto and Warren Roberts. Copyright © 1964, 1971 by Angelo Ravagli and C.M. Weekley, executors of the estate of Frieda Lawrence Ravagli. All rights reserved.

From "Love Was Once a Little Boy," in *Phoenix II: Uncollected, Unpublished, and Other Prose Works* by D.H. Lawrence. Copyright © 1959, 1963, 1968 by the Estate of Frieda Lawrence Ravagli.

From "We Need One Another," in *Phoenix: The Posthumous Papers of D. H. Lawrence.* Copyright 1936 by Frieda Lawrence. Renewed © 1964 by the estate of Frieda Lawrence Ravagli. All rights reserved.

HarperCollins books may be purchased for educational, business, or sales promotional use. For information please write: Special Markets Department, HarperCollins Publishers, Inc., 10 East 53rd Street, New York, NY 10022.

First HarperPerennial edition published 1991. Reissued in 1996.

Designed by Alma Orenstein

The Library of Congress has catalogued the hardcover edition as follows:

Welwood, John, 1943–
  Journey of the heart: intimate relationship and the path of love/John Welwood.—1st ed.
      p.   cm.
  Includes bibliographical references.
  ISBN 0-06-016475-1
  1. Marriage.   2. Interpersonal relations.   3. Intimacy (Psychology).   4. Love.   I. Title.
HQ734.W4845   1990
306.81—dc20   89-46563

ISBN 0-06-092742-9 (pbk.)
96 97 98 99 00 RRD 10 9 8 7 6 5 4 3

This book is dedicated to my teacher,
that warrior of all warriors,
the Dorje Dradul of Mukpo,
and to my wife and consort,
Jennifer,
both of whom, in their different ways,
have helped awaken my heart
and inspired my journey along the path.

Contents

For one human being to love another: that is perhaps the most difficult task of all . . . , the work for which all other work is but preparation. It is a high inducement to the individual to ripen . . . a great exacting claim upon us, something that chooses us out and calls us to vast things.

RAINER MARIA RILKE

Journey
OF THE
Heart

Introduction

> Be patient toward all that is unsolved in your heart
> and try to love the *questions themselves* like locked
> rooms or books that are written in a foreign
> tongue. The point is to live everything. *Live* the
> questions now. Perhaps you will then gradually,
> without noticing it, live your way some distant day
> into the answers.
>
> R. M. RILKE

NEVER BEFORE have intimate relationships called on us to face ourselves and each other with so much honesty and awareness. Maintaining an alive connection with an intimate partner today challenges us to free ourselves from old habits and blind spots and to develop the full range of our powers, sensitivities, and depths as human beings. In former times, if people wanted to explore the deeper mysteries of life, they would often enter the seclusion of a monastery or hermitage. For many of us today, however, intimate relationships have become the new wilderness that brings us face to face with all our gods and demons.

Since relationships can no longer be counted on as a predictable source of comfort or security, they bring us to a new crossroads, where we face a pivotal choice. We can struggle to hold on to wishful fantasies and old, outdated formulas, even though they neither match reality nor provide any useful directions. Or instead, we can learn to use the difficulties in our relationships as opportunities—to awaken and bring forth our finest human qualities, such as awareness, compassion, humor, wisdom, and a fearless dedication to truth. If we choose this approach, relationship becomes a path that can deepen our connection with ourselves and those we love and expand our sense of who we are.

THE LARGER PICTURE

In previous eras, family and society dictated the form and function of the man/woman relationship. Parents chose a child's marriage partner on the basis of family interests rather than the child's personal wishes. Since marriage was designed mainly to serve family and society, the quality of the personal relationship between husband and wife was of secondary importance. If a marriage was unhappy, community pressure would hold it together.

Only in the last few generations has this situation changed. Now that couples are increasingly removed from family, community, and widely shared values, there are few convincing *extrinsic* reasons for a man and a woman to sustain a life's journey together. Only the *intrinsic quality of their personal connection* can keep them going. Now, for the first time in history, every couple is on their own—to discover how to build a healthy relationship, and to forge their own vision of how and why to be together. *It is important to appreciate just how new this situation is. We are all pioneers in this unexplored territory.*

So rather than becoming discouraged, we could appreciate that we are trying to do something unique, which few societies have ever attempted, much less succeeded at—namely, to join romantic love, sexual passion, and a marriage of equals in a single, enduring relationship. Since men and women have rarely looked at each other eye to eye, as whole human beings, apart from roles, stereotypes, and inherited prescriptions, most couples through the ages have lived together without developing much personal intimacy. Nowadays, however, many of us seek a fuller kind of relatedness—mental, emotional, sexual, even spiritual—with our life partner. This means developing a whole new level of intimacy—by exploring and cultivating unrealized parts of ourselves in and through our connection with someone we love.

Developing this new level of intimacy in our relationships is both a personal and a collective imperative. It is an important step in healing the age-old rift between male and female and bringing together the two halves of our humanity. Centuries of imbalance between the masculine and feminine ways of being have left a deep wound in the human psyche. No one can escape the effects of this wound—which pervade both our inner and outer lives. Inwardly we experience it as a split between heart and mind, feeling and thinking, vulnerability and power; outwardly it manifests itself in the war between the sexes and in the ruthless exploitation of the earth that is endangering our whole planet. Until human consciousness can transform the ancient antagonism between masculine and feminine into a creative alliance, we will remain fragmented and at war with ourselves, as individuals, as couples, as societies, and as a race.

Our personal struggles to develop a deeper level of intimacy are a primary vehicle for this critical move forward that humanity needs to make. As we begin to move in this direction, the man/woman relationship takes on a larger purpose, beyond just survival or security: It becomes an instrument for the evolution of human consciousness. When we look at our personal difficulties with relationships in this light, they no longer seem so bewildering or overwhelming. For every evolutionary advance involves considerable trial and error before something new can emerge. If enough of us can rise to the current challenges of the man/woman relationship, using them as opportunities to peel away illusions, tap our deepest powers, and expand our sense of who we are, we can begin to develop the wisdom our age is lacking. We can give birth to a new vision of love and community that can help enlighten us as individuals and shape a new world in the process.[1]

CONSCIOUS RELATIONSHIP

Traditional marriage, based on social duty, and modern marriage, based more on hopes for perpetual romance and happiness, have both led to certain dead ends. What new ground can we find, beyond both hope and duty, to nourish and sustain a deeper, more satisfying love between men and women?

We can begin to cultivate a new spirit of engagement between the sexes by recognizing and welcoming the powerful opportunity that intimate relationships provide—to awaken to our deeper nature. Yet this also presents a tremendous challenge, for it means undertaking a journey in search of who we really are. Our connection with someone we love is one of the best vehicles for this journey. When we invite love to awaken us to the deeper powers of life, then working with its challenges becomes part of an ongoing adventure. *Intimacy becomes a path—* an unfolding process of discovery and revelation. *And relationship becomes, for the first time, conscious.*

The Greek myth of Eros and Psyche suggests what the journey of conscious relationship may entail. Eros becomes Psyche's lover on the condition that she must never attempt to see his face. He visits her by night, and for a while things go smoothly between them. But, never having seen her lover, Psyche begins to wonder who he really is. When she lights a lamp to see his face, he flies away, and she must undergo a series of trials to find him again. When she finally overcomes these trials, she is united with him again, only this time in a much fuller way, and their love can proceed in the light of day.

This myth points to the age-old separation between consciousness (Psyche) and love (Eros). Traditional Western marriages have been like love in the dark. Yet now that relationships no longer function smoothly in the old familiar grooves, they require a new kind of awareness. Like Psyche, we are presently undergoing the trials that every advance in consciousness entails.

BEGINNER'S MIND

Now that most of the old rules for relationships no longer apply, starting from "I don't know" is the essential first step on our *own* path of discovering what genuine intimacy, love, and communication involve. The Zen teacher Shunryu Suzuki Roshi called this act of putting aside opinions, beliefs, and preconceptions "beginner's mind." As he put it, "in the beginner's mind there are many possibilities, in the expert's, there are few." When we try to be experts at relationship—wanting always to stay in control or have it all together—we narrow our range of possibilities and play out old, predictable routines. Beginner's mind, by contrast, helps us open our awareness to whatever problem we are facing so we can ask essential questions that can spark new discoveries. In taking a fresh look at what is happening, we draw on the power of our creative intelligence, which alone can reveal new directions.

Our questions about how to love or how to make a relationship work only feel painful and irritating when we assume that we *should already have* the answers. Yet intimate relationships force us to face all the core issues of human existence—our family history; our personality dynamics; questions about who we are, how to communicate, how to handle our feelings, how to let love flow through us, how to be committed, how to let go and surrender. If relationships are difficult, it is because being human is difficult. So how could we know in advance how to make a relationship work? The question of how to be in a relationship is no other than the question of how to live.

Being human is always somewhat tenuous in that we know so little about how to *be*—how to be in this body, how to be on this earth, how to be authentically male or female, how to be fully alive. Intimate relationships, more than most areas of our lives, make us feel the rawness of these basic human questions, and thus compel us to explore more deeply who we are.

A NEW APPROACH

In my psychotherapy practice, I have found that when people demand instant answers before they have fully engaged with their questions, they are usually not yet ready to make real changes. I have also found that if I offer people solutions before they have this readiness, they never actually make use of them. That is why how-to books—unless they help people develop an inner readiness and willingness to change—are often ineffective. People read them, perhaps try out their techniques for a while, and soon forget them. Techniques rarely have any real impact when they are used as short-cuts, to bypass letting a difficulty affect us, work on us, and move us to find our own genuine response to it.

The most powerful agent of growth and transformation is something much more basic than any technique: a change of heart. This kind of inner shift can only happen when our questions or difficulties really touch us and arouse our willingness to approach things in a new way. Our problems may not disappear, but they become workable because we see them in a new context: Instead of feeling victimized by them, we find them calling on us to make important changes and grow in new directions. When our context shifts in this powerful, fundamental kind of way, it reveals paths across terrain that had previously seemed forbidding and impenetrable. Then the how-to's start to take care of themselves.

Most books on relationships take a problem-solving approach—pinpointing trouble spots and developing strategies to correct them. Like Western allopathic medicine, which focuses on relieving symptoms, that approach has a certain usefulness. However, for relationships to thrive in these difficult times, we need to go beyond mere symptom relief. Just as treating symptoms cannot in itself produce health, so solving problems is not enough to create healthy relationships. Instead of another set of problem-solving techniques, *we need a whole new approach to intimate relationships*—one that provides fresh vision and inspiration for working with love's challenges, by recognizing relationship as a path that can help us develop greater awareness, compassion, and spirit. Now that the old social and religious contexts have fallen away, this approach can provide a new context to guide us toward creating truly vital, healthy partnerships.

When we focus on problem-solving, we often imagine that if only we could get rid of the difficulties we are facing, if only we could just "get it right," *then* we could get on with having a happy relationship. However, since a relationship is always a living *process,* never a finished *product,* new questions and challenges continually arise. As soon as we handle one, another soon appears. If we can recognize that relationships, by their very nature, continually call on us to develop greater consciousness, then their difficulties are no longer just a nuisance; instead they can be seen as *an integral part of love's path.* For they compel us to bring the light of awareness to the dark, unconscious parts of ourselves and mobilize inner resources—such as patience, generosity, kindness, and bravery—that give us a larger, deeper sense of who we are.

So instead of trying to ward off the challenging questions that relationships pose, we need to let them work on us, like an inoculation. This is more like homeopathic medicine, which works by subtly intensifying a symptom in order to activate the organism's natural healing response. Though our questions may be irritating at first, as they work on us they stimulate our creative intelligence, triggering larger healing, transformative powers within us and thus fortifying our system as a whole. This is what will provide the strength and courage to keep moving forward on love's path, regardless of the difficulties we encounter.

Thus opening more deeply to our questions is the essential ground of relationship as a path. Honoring the "I don't know" instead of fighting it can help us discover new possibilities and resources—right in the midst of whatever problem we are facing. This gives us a way of starting fresh again and again, whether we have been single most of our lives or married for twenty years.

Of course, acknowledging our uncertainty brings up anxiety in the face of the unknown. We feel much safer when we think we have all the answers. But love between the sexes is, of all things, *not safe*. Intimate relationships are not safe! That is not their nature. They unmask and expose us, and bring us face to face with life in all its power and mystery, through contact with what is most different from us—an *other*. Unless we are willing to explore the unknown in ourselves, in the other, and in the relations between us, we will never advance very far along the path of love.

At first it seems unsettling to discover that love has no easy solution, that there is no simple remedy for the rawness of the heart that loving someone deeply opens up. Yet once we give up seeking an easy way out, an important shift can take place. Love's rough edges can become a powerful resource, for they connect us more fully with our heart—that larger source of intelligence that *can* guide us through all the uncertainties and complexities of relationship. Through cultivating a taste for our rawness—which has a sweetness all its own—we invite our heart to show us the way.

PART I

The Nature of Path

1

Intimate Relationship as a Practice and a Path

> It furthers one to have somewhere to go . . .
>
> *I CHING*

> We need a path, not to go from here to there, but to go from here to here.
>
> JAKUSHO KWONG

THE SPANISH PHILOSOPHER Ortega y Gasset once wrote that "no land in human topography is less explored than love." If this be so, then the dream of love current in our society—which tells us that finding the right person, falling in love, and settling down together is the ticket to everlasting bliss and security—is like a tourist's approach to this unknown land. This fantasy leads us to believe that relationships should somehow unfold in predictable ways and require little special effort or attention. As the Beatles sang: "All you need is love . . . it's easy." Yet just as going abroad to "do" the familiar sights on a packaged tour limits perception and diminishes the joy of making new discoveries, so when we try to make relationships fit into a familiar, conventional fantasy we lose the spice that brings out the richest flavors of love: the unknown.

Real intimacy is, first and foremost, a journey into this unknown. Relating to an *other* of the *other* sex faces us with the great other inside us as well—a whole range of unexplored qualities and dimensions of our being, beyond the familiar "me" we know so well. In confronting us with the great unknown inside us, love sharpens our senses and calls on us to grow and develop in unforeseen ways.

So to taste the real depth and richness of love's potential, we need to explore this uncharted territory on our own rather than follow tourist maps. Trying to make a relationship match some fixed image in our mind works against developing our deepest resources, which grow out of responding to the real challenges along the way. What we most need today is not some ideal goal to live up to, but a sense of the real adventure on which we are embarking. The *dream of love* distracts us from the real *path of love,* which continually leads into vast, unforeseen possibilities.

Path is a term that points to the great challenge of human existence: the need to awaken, each in our own way, to the greater possibilities that life presents. The nature of a path is to lead us on a journey, and it is life's deepest urge to move forward in this way. Whenever our lives have this sense of forward momentum, we feel an unmistakable stream of vitality flowing through us, which tells us that we are on to something real. Unfortunately, however, we are often not aligned with this force moving deep within. As the Sufi poet Rumi described our situation, "We who are blind think our horse is lost, yet all the while he is sweeping us onward like the wind." Though the steed of our aliveness is carrying us forward whether we like it or not, we often remain asleep in the saddle.

Thus relationships can proceed in either of two directions—toward sleep or wakefulness—and we each have a personal choice about which way they will go. We can try to use them to prop us up, to allay our insecurities, or to prove that we are worthwhile, acceptable, lovable. Doubting that we are basically good to begin with, we may seek comfort and consolation from them. We may even try to turn them into a fortress against impermanence, to protect us from the ever-changing nature of life. Yet when we use relationships primarily for comfort and security, they only stagnate, putting us more deeply asleep and reinforcing habitual patterns of fear and self-doubt.

The other choice is to regard intimacy as a way to come more fully alive, by helping us bring forth *the goodness and strength already present within us.* Instead of looking to a relationship for shelter, we could welcome its power to wake us up in those areas where we are asleep and where we avoid naked, direct contact with life. This approach puts us on a path. It commits us to movement and change, providing forward direction by showing us exactly where we most need to grow. Embracing relationship as a path also gives us a practice: learning to use each difficulty along the way as an opportunity to go further, to connect more deeply, not just with our partner, but with our own aliveness as well.

By contrast, dreaming that love will save us, solve all our problems or provide a steady state of bliss or security only keeps us stuck in wishful fantasy, undermining the real power of love—which is to transform us. For our relationships to flourish, we need to see them in a new way—as a series of opportunities for developing greater awareness, discovering deeper truth, and becoming more fully human.

CONFLICT AS OPPORTUNITY

Unfortunately, not many couples are prepared to take the adventurous route, to make use of the challenges that their love holds in store for them. Yet when this kind of shift in perspective does occur, it points the way toward a richer and more deeply satisfying relationship.

One couple I worked with had been happily married for two years without having to face any major challenges in their relationship. Then, during a series of arguments over their children from previous marriages, they hurt each other deeply. The woman, Allyn, had never been able to deal with difficult feelings. Her way of handling her hurt and vulnerability when she felt badly treated by her husband was to explode in rage and then withdraw. This would cause Matthew, a lawyer who approached everything logically, to close down as well. By the time they came to see me for counseling, they had reached a complete standoff and were barely on speaking terms.

At first they wanted me to "fix it" for them—provide some advice or solution that would help them put their relationship back the way it was. But it was too late for that. They disagreed on too many core issues and had hurt each other too deeply to go back to their old patterns of avoidance and denial. Instead, their conflict presented them with an opportunity to grow and evolve. Allyn was being called on to open to her tender, vulnerable feelings instead of avoiding them through rage and blame. As for Matthew, facing the rawness he felt with his wife provided perhaps the greatest chance he would ever have to open to a deeper dimension of life. What else in his fast-paced world would call on him so powerfully to soften up, accept his own tender feelings, and expose his heart to the light of day? It was inspiring to work with this couple as they gradually came to realize that saving their relationship meant breaking through old limitations and growing in significant new ways.

This kind of growth is challenging because it often costs us what we hold most dear: namely, our old ways of staying secure and defended. Yet the promise in such a situation is equally powerful: If we open up in the ways it requires, our relationship will deepen immeasurably. And we will broaden out as human beings, becoming more flexible, loving, and responsive to life as a whole.

BECOMING FULLY HUMAN

When we welcome the opportunities they provide for growth, relationships become a powerful force in our development, providing just the kind of impetus we need if we are to realize our larger potential. As human beings we are the "unfinished animal." Our nature is open-ended and malleable, and we are forever discovering anew what we are capable of. Although we are given a human body at birth, we are not given our full humanity. *Becoming human means discovering our fullness and learning to live from it. This involves bringing forth more of who we really are and becoming more available to whatever life presents.*

To live from our fullness, we must have access to a whole range of human capacities. We need power, fierceness, and toughness to persevere and get things done; compassion, tenderness, gentleness, and generosity to nurture ourselves and those we love. We must be able to feel both joy and sorrow if we are to taste life's many flavors. We need patience and determination, as well as humor and abandon. Sometimes we need to exert discipline; other situations call for letting go into sensuality and playfulness. We need both discriminating intellect and spontaneous intuition. We must be able to act decisively when necessary. At other times the most powerful thing is simply to let things be.

All the most universally valued qualities—humor, generosity, gentleness, courage, patience, and so on—help us realize and express our humanness, by enabling us *to be fully present with what is.* Generosity, for instance, allows us to extend ourselves to what is going on around us, while patience enables us to let it be. Tenderness is a willingness to be pierced by reality, while fierceness allows us to cut through and penetrate situations. Humor is a way of playing with what is, taking it lightly, rather than making it solid and heavy. Each of these qualities allows us to engage with a different facet of reality. The more of them we have access to, the more we can embrace the whole of life—in its joys and delights, as well as in its difficulties and sorrows.

Each of us has access to this whole spectrum of human qualities, at least as seed potentials. Yet most of us have developed one sort of quality—such as toughness—while neglecting its opposite—such as tenderness. In this way, we are all somewhat lopsided and incomplete. This sense of incompleteness is what draws us toward relationship. Yet what would complete us? Is it just companionship? Beyond finding companionship, we have a deeper need to live from our fullness, to engage with life as fully as we can. What we are missing is the other half of our human wholeness—those untapped potentials that need to be cultivated if we are to realize the full range and depth of who we are.

Our longing to taste life fully is what sets us on a path. This longing arises from a larger intelligence operating in us, which leads us toward those qualities we most need to realize. Thus we are often most strongly attracted to people who manifest qualities we lack or who challenge us to develop them. We feel excitement and passion when we sense that such a person could help us realize a greater fullness and depth of being than we have yet discovered. Thus falling in love is born out of our yearning to come into ourselves more fully.

Yet if we are blind to this larger intelligence operating in us, imagining instead that someone else could give us what we lack, then our passion may bring us more pain than enrichment. For instance, if a man imagines that he can find the spontaneity and aliveness missing from his life only through vivacious women, his relationships with them may only intensify his hunger and emptiness. Yet if he can discover in his attractions to such women a desire to realize his own fiery, energetic qualities, then he has a path.

CONDITIONED PATTERNS

What prevents us from living more fully and having more enriching relationships is a set of narrow, limited notions about who we are. It takes dedication and exertion to break out of these constricting ideas. Whether our seed potentials ripen and bear fruit depends entirely on whether we cultivate them and remove the obstacles to their growth.

Yet by the time we start to become aware that we have such a choice, a great deal of heavy baggage already encumbers us. We have become conditioned into habitual reaction patterns that cloud our awareness, distort our feelings, and restrict our capacity to open to life and to love. The seed of our humanity has become encased in a hard shell. Our defensive postures, which we originally fashioned to shield us from pain, have become a dead weight keeping us from bursting forth into life's radiance. Since these old ways of doing things fight for dear life to maintain their hold on us, it takes intention and effort to break loose from their grip.

We have no single word in English for these conditioned defensive patterns, so I will borrow a term from the Eastern traditions—*karma,* which literally means "the action of cause and effect." Although this term as used in the East often refers to inherited tendencies from past lives, we can also use it in a more psychological sense to describe conditioned tendencies established during *this* life, from childhood through the present. Regardless of where we think of karma as coming from, the result is the same: years of habitual contraction, avoidance, denial, unconsciousness, and fear have entangled us in a web of reactive patterns, threatening to constrict or cut off our life force.

HEART AND KARMA

Yet underneath all our conditioning, the basic nature of the human heart is an awake presence, *an openness to reality.* We are born curious, responsive, and alert to the world around us. As Thoreau put it, "Be it life or death, we crave only reality"—and this taste for reality points to a basic sanity and wholesomeness at the core of our nature. Our innate sensitivity and desire to connect with reality is the seed of wisdom, which can ripen within each one of us. Unfortunately, the accumulated inertia of the past, as it has become frozen into our personality structure, usually prevents our larger "wisdom mind" or "wisdom heart" from fully ripening. T. S. Eliot points to this other side of us when he writes, in contrast to Thoreau, "human kind cannot bear very much reality."

So each of us has two forces at work inside us: an embryonic wisdom that wants to blossom from the depths of our being, and the imprisoning weight of our karma; an unconditioned awake presence that wants to connect fully with life, and our conditioned personality patterns that narrow our perception and keep us half-asleep. From birth to death, these two forces are always at work, and our lives hang in the balance. In youth, our green life energy is usually stronger than our habitual patterns. We are still flexible, our habits have not totally solidified, and we imagine that we can overcome any obstacles standing in our way. Yet every time we repeat a habitual reaction, we wear "grooves" in our psyche. By the time we reach old age, these grooves have become deeply etched. Old people who have not worked on themselves become inflexible, stuck, set in their ways. Somewhere in midlife the weight of karmic accumulation starts to overpower our life force. Midlife crisis is the realization that time is running out and our karma is catching up with us. At that point, we can no longer just get by on our youthful energy. Unless we bring our larger intelligence and awareness to bear on our defensive postures, they will harden further, freezing us into a living rigor mortis. This cannot be emphasized too strongly: If we do nothing, our karma *will bury us.*

Intimate relationships can help free us from our conditioning by allowing us to see exactly how and where we are stuck. They continually bring us up against things in ourselves that we cannot stand. They stir up all our worst fears and neuroses—in living Technicolor. When we live alone, we are often unaware of our habitual patterns because we live inside them. A relationship, on the other hand, heightens our awareness of all our rough edges. When someone we love reacts to our neurotic patterns, they bounce back on us and we can no longer ignore them. As we see and feel the ways we are stuck, a desire to move in a new direction naturally begins to stir in us. There is ferment, and thus a real possibility for change and renewal. Our path begins to unfold.

Unfortunately, many couples lose heart when their initial honeymoon period comes to an end and they start to encounter difficult things in themselves and each other. Yet as long as we imagine that something is wrong when a relationship stirs up our most difficult emotional issues, we will never be able to set forth on love's real journey. In my experience, the greatest obstacle to growth in a relationship is a couple's belief that "it shouldn't be this hard." Yet the reason it often *is* hard is that we are set in our ways, and it takes great energy and dedication to break free of them. Love helps us to do so, by inspiring us to open our heart. The honeymoon phase in a relationship is a pure experience of open heart. It gives us a sense of what is possible, which we can draw on for inspiration when we bog down. Trying to maintain that state, however, only prevents us from moving forward.

When Matthew and Allyn's honeymoon phase ended and they began to discover the real difficulties in their relationship, they at first felt bewildered and discouraged. For they had no idea how or even why they should proceed with a relationship if it brought up so much pain. Matthew's struggle with Allyn was calling on him to come to terms with what he feared most—his own feelings. He had long ago decided to cut himself off from them and become completely logical instead, so that he would never have to be like his mother, whom he regarded as "an emotional wreck." Yet now he was face to face with all his wife's feelings, and—what was worse!—his own as well. As for Allyn, she had worked hard never to feel needy and vulnerable again after years of neglect as a child. Yet these were the exact feelings that her struggle with Matthew aroused.

From the standpoint of bliss or security, this couple appeared to be in terrible shape. Yet their situation also awakened them to an important new realization—that their love was asking each of them to grow and their conflict was showing them the directions in which they most needed to go. From a path point of view, their difficulties provided a tremendous opportunity, by motivating them to clear out obstacles in the way of their development. This new perspective gave them the vision and incentive they needed in order to persevere through this difficult period in their relationship.

Intimate relationships are ideally suited as a path *because they inspire our heart to open while at the same time activating all the pain and confusion of our karmic entanglements.* If anyone else but Allyn had challenged Matthew to face his feelings, he might have simply disappeared. But since his heart was so open to her, he could not get away that easily! Because he loved his wife and wanted to be with her, he had to go forth and confront his greatest fears.

Love is a transformative power precisely because it brings the two different sides of ourselves—the expansive and the contracted, the awake and the asleep—into direct contact. Our heart begins to work on our karma: Rigid places in us that we have hidden from view suddenly come out in the open, and soften in love's blazing warmth. And our karma starts to work on our heart: As we come up against difficult places in ourselves and our partner, our heart has to open and expand in new ways. In this way, the challenges of intimate relationship provide a rare and special opportunity—to venture beyond our self-imposed limitations and claim the larger power and wisdom that is our human birthright.

2

Warrior of the Heart

What now seems to you opaque, you will make
transparent with your blazing heart . . .

R. M. RILKE

AS OUR LOVE FOR ANOTHER PERSON brings our heart into contact
with our karma, stirring up feelings of uncertainty, confusion,
fear, or vulnerability, it reveals a certain rawness at the core of
our experience. Normally we try to manage and manipulate our
lives to avoid this feeling, which seems to threaten our security
or identity. Yet this rawness is central to our humanity—we
simply become more aware of it when we love. Letting ourselves
feel it can soften us and loosen up old, rigid patterns. Therefore
it is an important key to our growth.

We are raw in two senses: Our experience is, at its core, not
only tender and sensitive, but also basically "uncooked." Because we are the "unfinished animal," our experience is never
fully formed, polished, complete. We are a mix of wildly different impulses and energies, many of which do not fit together
smoothly. Our feelings never quite fit into any nice, neat pack-
ages or measure up to our ideal image of how we think they
should be. To be at ease with ourselves, we need to learn to trust
this rawness at the core of our experience, and move freely with
it, perhaps even celebrate it.

This means learning to accept our experience *as it is,* instead of trying to make it match some preconceived image. *To*

be fully present to our experience as it is, without shrinking or turning away from it, is to be a warrior—of the heart. Being a warrior in this sense does not mean acting aggressively or "toughing it out." It means prevailing through inner strength rather than through domination, as exemplified in the ancient Eastern dictum "The greatest warrior is one who never has to use his sword." This approach is more like practicing *aikido,* a nonaggressive martial art that involves moving, almost dancing, *with* what comes to us rather than pitting ourselves *against* it. To be a warrior of the heart means welcoming whatever arises in relationships, no matter how difficult or challenging, as an opportunity to grow stronger, to call forth new inner resources.

Approaching the difficulties of relationship in this warrior spirit—as steps along a path, as movements in a dance, rather than as a nuisance or a threat—cuts through our habitual tendency to contract into an oppositional stance when something threatens us. This can help us relate to ourselves and others in a fuller, more compassionate and wakeful way.

What will allow us to stay present in the face of whatever is going on around us? To draw on our warrior spirit, we need to find a source of strength inside ourselves, by developing a deeper relationship with our own being. In particular, we need to cultivate three essential capacities that enable us to be with what is—awareness, courage, and gentleness.

AWARENESS: CLEARLY SEEING WHAT IS

The most basic quality of a warrior is awareness. The more awareness we have, the more skillfully we can handle whatever arises. Awareness is by far the most essential, powerful resource we have for effecting change and working with life's challenges. That is why the samurai in ancient Japan often studied meditation, the practice of mindful awareness—seeing simply and directly what is happening from moment to moment.

Usually when we say, "I am aware that . . . ," we are stating what we know, rather than practicing pure awareness. Awareness is much greater than knowledge or thought. It is the activity of our larger intelligence, which responds immediately to what is, before we draw on any concept to analyze or interpret it. Its basic nature is *clarity*. Certain meditative traditions liken awareness to a mirror, which reflects without bias. It has also been likened to the sun, which illumines whatever it shines upon. Awareness radiates a broad, diffuse light that can reveal what is going on in any situation, beyond any idea we have about it.

Another important feature of awareness is its *fluidity*. Like a zoom lens, it can move back from any state of mind or emotion we are caught in, so that we can gain a larger perspective on what is happening. It can also penetrate situations, zeroing in on their subtlest details.

A third characteristic of awareness is its *stability* and *continuity*. No matter how much our thoughts or emotions carry us away, at any moment we can always return to being present and simply noticing what is happening. No matter how difficult a situation may be, when we face it squarely, letting our awareness shine forth and clarify what is happening, we "find our seat"; that is, we regain balance and confidence. When thoughts take control, they cause us to lose our seat and feel disconnected. When we practice simple awareness, however, we can keep our seat and go forth to meet what is in front of us in a saner way. The classic meditation posture—sitting still with an upright posture—both expresses and supports this stability of awareness.

Cultivating this clear, fluid, and flexible awareness enables us to confront whatever arises. Such an awareness can be practiced right in the midst of our relationships. Let us take a simple example, one that everyone has experienced: My partner has said something that has hurt me and touched off a fight. At first, I am caught up in feeling hurt—my body aches and my mind is swarming with painful thoughts and associations. I don't like to feel this way, so I start to react against it. Yet my pain is like the famous tar baby in the Uncle Remus tale: The more I struggle with it, the more I become entangled and stuck in it. I start to tell myself stories that only intensify my pain: "She'll never understand me," "She likes to attack me, she's too aggressive,"

"Maybe this relationship is finished," "I don't know how to make her happy." Each of these stories touches off further reactions in me, and the more I get caught up in my reactions, the more I lose touch with what is really happening.

If I plug into the story—"She likes to attack me, that's just the way she is"—I may then do something to get back at her or I may decide to close myself off to her. Yet both these defensive reactions only complicate the situation further because they are not accurate responses to what is really going on. To find out what *is* going on, I must put aside my stories and bring some fresh awareness to the situation.

To regain awareness, I need to take a step back from the whirlwind of my reactions. Although this may take some practice at first, it is always possible because the nature of awareness is mobile and fluid. Instead of continuing to be tossed around in turbulent thoughts and emotions, I can let my awareness move back from them, like a zoom lens in reverse, and simply acknowledge the whole pain I am feeling. When I can do this, it is as though I step out of a blazing fire that is consuming me, and sit down next to it instead.

Once I create some space for myself, I am no longer trapped in the fire's flames. I can then allow the fire to be there as it is, without having to resist it. I still feel its heat, but it no longer burns me alive. In other words, when I can make space for my hurt to be there, and when I can be present with my awareness "next to it," "on the edge of it," I find my seat. This brings relief. I am no longer stuck in an oppositional struggle. Instead, I have more *clarity*—I can simply recognize that I am hurting, without becoming so embroiled in a drama around it. I have more *freedom* of movement because I am not caught in reacting against the pain. And in taking my seat, I feel more *stability* and strength.

Having made space for my pain and regained my awareness in this way, I can then face the pain more directly. Without trying to "make something out of it," I can sit with it in a spirit of inquiry. Although my mind may provide plenty of stories about why I feel so bad, in truth, *I don't really know* why I am hurting so much right now or what I need to do next. Instead of trying to figure things out with my mind, I can look into the pain for clues. Letting my awareness penetrate the pain in a gently questioning way, I can inquire into it ("What's really hurting so much right now?") and listen to what the feeling might have to tell me.

As I do this, I begin to see that my partner's words touched a part of me that I have a hard time dealing with, one that I would rather not have to acknowledge at all. So, as it turns out, the real issue isn't that my partner is too aggressive; it's that I feel so vulnerable when anyone sees this part of me. Now that I have penetrated to the core of the matter through mobilizing my awareness, I am no longer in danger of reacting foolishly and making the situation worse. Things can begin to move forward because I am in touch with what is true for me. This also allows me to communicate more effectively. Instead of being defensive and reactive, I can share with her how hard it is to let her see this part of me. When I do this, she softens, and we are back in the flow of our connectedness again. In this way, we can always find a way forward when we regain our awareness and actively bring it to bear on whatever situation we are in.

While becoming aware of what is happening is simple enough, it is of course not always easy to do. This is because we have an investment in maintaining and promoting an old familiar *version* of reality, and this prevents us from seeing what is actually going on. Especially in the area of love, we are blinded by conditioned hopes and fears, by cherished preconceptions, beliefs, and opinions of all kinds, both personal and collective.

We perpetuate these conditioned ways of perceiving the world through repetitive stories we tell ourselves about "the way things are." These kinds of stories are mental fabrications, judgments or interpretations that put what is happening into a familiar framework. Usually we do not recognize these stories as our own invention; instead, we believe that they represent reality. Stories often operate in the background of the mind, as part of an ongoing stream of subconscious gossip that we keep up with ourselves. The less conscious we are of how they control us, the more they keep us locked into old patterns of behavior. The greatest obstacles in relationships are often our stories about how we think relationships should be. ("If you love someone, you should always keep them happy . . . you should always want to be there . . . you should set aside your anger.") They narrow our options and keep us stuck in very tight boxes.

This dense fabric of entrenched beliefs, stories, and reaction patterns acts as a filter that clouds and obscures the natural clarity and fluidity of awareness. Because this web is so thick and entangling, we need to find ways to catch ourselves in the act of constructing these stories, see through them, and return to a basic, simple awareness of what is immediately happening. We need to discover that we can, at any moment, make a shift from thought to awareness, which is the larger space in which thoughts and stories arise. So, just as practicing a musical instrument allows us to play more fluidly, we must at first intentionally *practice* awareness before it can flow more fluidly and reflect more accurately on its own. In the Zen tradition, this is called "polishing the mirror." With greater consciousness, we can begin to dislodge the stories controlling our behavior, thus developing greater clarity and freedom in our life.

The example I've just given on dealing with pain illustrates how we can begin to practice awareness in the midst of everyday life situations. This is the approach I generally take in my psychotherapy practice. (It is related to the Focusing method, developed by Eugene Gendlin.)[1] An even more thorough, far-reaching method of cultivating awareness and seeing through the whole storytelling function of the mind is the practice of mindfulness meditation. Since it is difficult to practice awareness when we are suddenly beset by the emotional crosscurrents of relationship conflicts, a regular meditation practice can be especially helpful. It can teach us how to step out of the tangle of our emotions and stories, and relate more directly to what is actually happening.

Mindfulness practice involves sitting up straight, following the breath, and noticing our thoughts and perceptions, then letting them go and returning to a state of simple presence. Instead of trying to restrain the conditioned mind or force it to be a certain way, this practice provides plenty of space in which the mind can play out its dramas. We begin to witness how we are continually making up stories about who we are, what we are doing, and what will happen next. At other times, we discover a wider, deeper quality of ongoing awareness, which is clear, fluid, and continuous like a steady stream flowing underneath all our various states of mind. This contrast helps us make an important distinction—between our immediate experience and our interpretations of that experience. We start to cultivate a healthy skepticism toward the storytelling aspect of mind and develop a more discriminating awareness.

Through this kind of practice we can learn to be more present with whatever is happening in our experience, just as it is, from moment to moment, apart from our beliefs, judgments, and fantasies about it. This helps us connect with our own living wisdom and "keep our seat," so that we do not always get thrown or carried away by the mind's inventions. Drawing on this keener, more flexible kind of awareness can help us avoid becoming bogged down in the heavy emotional dramas that intimate relationships often set in motion.

COURAGE: CONNECTING WITH WHAT IS

Once we start to develop greater awareness of what is happening in a relationship, however, we may not like what we see. As we see our flaws, our partner's shortcomings, or various imperfections in the relationship itself, difficult feelings arise. Having seen what is, we may doubt that we can handle it, and become tempted to avert our gaze and fall back into unconsciousness.

So it is not enough just to see what is happening; we must also be willing to extend ourselves, to make a connection with it. This means opening ourselves to our experience and *feeling* it, facing it squarely and letting it affect us. Being courageous does not mean that we will not feel afraid. Rather, it is a willingness to stay open to our fear and rawness, without rigidifying or running away. In the meditation posture, an upright spine, head, and shoulders express this quality of bravery—looking straight ahead without collapsing or curling in on ourselves.

When we practice awareness, we also cultivate courage, for awareness actually contains courage in it. To wake up and confront what is actually happening, rather than just going along with old stories and reaction patterns, *is* an act of bravery. In our example, courage appears when I am willing to "sit on the edge of my pain" and look at it face to face. We can learn to do the same with fear, anger, grief, or any other state of mind. We can move out to the edge of the fear, take our seat there, and inquire into it instead of being controlled by our fear stories (e.g., "If I tell the truth, she'll leave," "If she leaves, I can't go on living.") and the further panic they generate.

When we connect with our experience, we also cultivate our being—our ability *to be* in the present moment. This allows us to feel our heart. The word *courage* derives from *coeur,* the French word for "heart." Thus the essence of courage is being willing to feel our heart even in situations that are difficult or painful.

GENTLENESS: MAKING FRIENDS WITH WHAT IS

In courageously facing what is happening in our relationships, we inevitably come up against feelings we dislike or would rather not have—such as pain, disappointment, fear, insecurity, anger, or jealousy. So it is not enough just to practice courage. To stay connected with our being and to remain fluid and flexible when we come up against obstacles, we must also be gentle with ourselves.

Since real intimacy always leads into unknown territory, we find our way only through trial and error. As we leave behind old, familiar ways of being and move toward new states of balance, falling into one extreme or another is unavoidable along the way. This is how we grow. So we must give ourselves permission to go overboard sometimes. If we attack ourselves for going off course, we cannot learn from mistakes and use them as part of our path. Therefore cultivating gentleness with ourselves is essential for fostering inner growth and development.

Practicing gentleness does not mean always liking what we see or simply tolerating whatever goes on in a relationship. If we don't like our feelings, we can make room for our dislike as well. If we're angry about a situation, we can let our anger be there too. Whatever arises, we can learn to be with it and *let it be* as it is. When we open to our experience as it is, without imposing any blame or manipulation on it, we start to make friends with ourselves. Only then can our defensive structures begin to relax, clearing the way for our larger wisdom to shine through and guide us.

Like courage, gentleness is contained within awareness. For awareness holds no grudge or bias—like the sun, it simply allows us to see what is. If courage is the side of awareness that faces things directly, gentleness is the side that accommodates or makes space for what is there. The act of surrounding whatever we are feeling with awareness, no matter how terrible we *think* it is, is a very friendly thing to do.

TAKING STEPS FORWARD

Awareness, courage, and gentleness are the basic "weapons" of the warrior of the heart. They cut through our habitual tendencies to fight or flee when we come up against painful or difficult situations. In this way, they allow us to convert whatever challenges we are facing into stepping-stones in our development.

Yet most of us, if we carry these weapons at all, have let them become dull from lack of use. Fortunately, that does not disqualify us from venturing forth on love's path. For relationships provide many hard surfaces on which to sharpen these abilities. And the sharper they become, the farther we can advance along this path.

We all face certain obstacles that stand in the way of having a healthy, fulfilling relationship. We may doubt that we are lov-

able. We may never feel ready to make a commitment. Or perhaps we can never find the "right one" for us. Typically such
impasses cause us to swing between hope—that we will somehow be rescued from our situation—and despair—that we are
somehow defective or doomed. Yet telling ourselves stories like
"Something is wrong with me, this shouldn't be happening,"
only keeps us from seeing the immediate stepping-stones right
in front of us.

Instead, if we can let our difficulties with intimacy touch us,
they will show us what we most need to work on to come into
deeper relationship with ourselves and with others. When we let
ourselves feel the rawness these difficulties bring up, we start to
get in touch with deeper powers—our capacities to be present
with whatever is happening and to find a way to work with it. In
this way, whatever seems most impossible about relationships,
whatever problem, question, or confusion we have—if we see it,
feel it, go toward it, *use* it—*is* our path.

To call upon our warrior spirit and use love's difficulties as
path, we can always begin by asking of the difficulty, "What is
this pointing to in me that I need to look at?" Every obstacle or
challenge that we face contains an implicit question, which can
help us find a new direction. *Questions are an invitation to greater
awareness.* They point us toward areas of our experience that
need our attention. So when we make the question that is implicit in our difficulty explicit, we are inviting our awareness to
enter the situation and guide us.

When we address our impasse in this way, we can use it to
generate useful "path questions" for ourselves: "What is this
difficulty pointing to? What is it trying to teach me? What can
I learn from this situation?" The point of asking such questions
is not to come up with an immediate answer. When we try too
hard to find an answer, our busy conditioned mind takes over
and we only become more confused. But if we can take these
questions deep inside us, using them to help us explore neglected areas of our experience, they will point us in new directions.

One woman, in considering why her prospective partners

never worked out for her, discovered in herself a strong underground fear of men, as well as a distrust of her own femininity. Thus she realized that her difficulty in finding the right man pointed to some major conflicts about intimacy that she needed to resolve. In her childhood, love had become associated with guilt, debt, and pain. To be loved meant giving herself up. As long as she held that deeply ingrained belief, she was not really ready for the kind of relationship she longed for.

It took courage for this woman to bring these issues to light and deal with them. Yet painful as this was, it felt much better than remaining stuck in hope or despair. For it gave her a direction: She needed to find her own power and resolve her old fears of love before she could truly give herself to a man. Instead of complaining "Why is this happening to me?" she could start to relate to her situation more actively.

Realizing that her impasse with men was helping her take an important step forward in her development also allowed her to be more gentle with herself about her situation. Instead of blaming herself for not having a man, she began to give herself space and time to develop in new ways—to go deep within, face her tendency to give men magical power over her, and eventually find her own light which she could trust. Connecting with herself in this deeper way also helped her appreciate herself as a woman. As she expanded and filled out, she no longer expected men to fill her gaps, and she became more interested in them for who they really were. Consequently, more interesting men started appearing in her life and finding her attractive.

Thus bringing awareness, courage, and gentleness to bear on stuck and impossible areas of relationship ignites the intrinsic wisdom of the heart, which can burn through old patterns of denial and avoidance. If our heart is like a flame, our karmic obstructions are the fuel that this fire needs in order to blaze brightly. Although the burning up of old karma creates great turbulence, it also releases tremendous energy. As our habitual patterns start to break down, we gain access to a fuller spectrum of our human qualities.

So instead of trying to hide the places where we feel raw or confused, fearing that they will spoil the romance, we can, as warriors, actually invite them to come up and burn in love's fire. This allows us to discover that we have access to greater depth and power than we ever imagined. As the flame of the heart burns brighter, consuming our conditioned patterns, our confusions, and our fears, it generates warmth and lights our way.

We cannot become warriors of the heart overnight. Only through practice in working with love's challenges can our being start to unfold, step by step. This gradual unfolding is the path quality of love. Such a path does not lead anywhere except to the heart of our humanness. Love has no other goal. The path is the goal.

3

Joining Heaven and Earth

To enter into an intimate relationship is to be swept up in a play of self and other, a ceaseless dance of shifting polarities. The most basic polarity in relationship—the tension between our separateness as individuals and our desire to connect with another—is set in motion as soon as we find ourselves attracted to someone. Suddenly we want to burst forth and open ourselves to this person who moves and touches us in ways we barely comprehend. Yet at the same time we may hesitate and hang back, holding on for dear life to the very separateness we also long to overcome.

At the core of our existence, we all experience the basic ache of feeling separate. We long to be united with someone or something outside of ourselves, so that we do not have to feel this ache so sharply. So when we finally find someone we feel close to, it may seem like a kind of salvation—no longer must we wander this lonely world all by ourselves. Yet in satisfying our urge to merge, it is all too easy to become *sub*merged in a relationship, waking up one day to realize that we have lost something essential—ourself!

Relationships always involve this kind of fluctuation between bonding with another and maintaining our integrity as individuals, yielding to our partner and asserting ourselves, reaching out and going deep within. It is not surprising that so many couples lose the flow and rhythm of this dance, falling out of step and winding up deadlocked in antagonistic positions. Moving smoothly and gracefully between such opposite poles is not an easy thing to do, for it calls on us to develop and integrate very different sides of our nature.

Giving ourselves to a loving partnership while remaining true to ourselves, learning to balance "we" and "me," is the central challenge of intimate relationships. In helping us learn this dance, relationships teach us to come to terms with a basic duality at the core of our existence. Being human involves joining, or marrying, two very different tendencies at work inside us. On one hand, we need to discover our individual path in this life, connect deeply with ourselves, and honor our own truth. On the other hand, we also need to loosen our preoccupation with ourselves, let go into life, and connect with something larger, beyond ourselves.

These two needs arise from two different sides of our nature, which exert opposite pulls on us. In larger cosmic terms, human life unfolds on the edge where heaven and earth meet. Our very posture—feet firmly planted on the ground and head raised toward the open sky—perfectly depicts our twofold nature. Since we are creatures of this earth, we have no choice but to be right here, right where we are at this point in time and space. We cannot escape the determining influences of our personal conditioning, our desires and feelings, our history and karma. At the same time our upright head and shoulders enable us to see far-off things—horizons, stars, suns, planets, and the infinite reaches of space all around. We also belong to this vastness.

Half of our life is about taking our seat on this earth, and creating structures (such as home, family, work) that further our unfolding. This forces us to accept and make use of the personal circumstances we are given to work with. No matter how grand our hopes, dreams, or visions, putting them into practice always involves grappling with the limitations of our culture, our body and personal history, and our emotional temperament.

The other half of life involves surrendering to what is beyond us, letting go of the structures we have created, and continually moving forward into new, unknown areas. The heaven principle working in us calls on us to expand, develop larger vision, and explore greater possibilities, beyond what we already know or see right in front of us. This use of the term *heaven* is not meant to conjure up an image of some higher realm above or apart from this world. Instead, it indicates the way in which the human spirit is vast and open like the sky, never entirely encompassed by personality, the limitations of conditioning, or the constraints of form and matter.

HEAVENLY INSPIRATION

When we fall in love, we get a powerful glimpse of the heaven principle in action. My longing to taste the larger life beyond me makes me feel inspired by another being and delight in the ways she is different from me. *Inspire* literally means "to breathe in." The spark of inspiration is like a breath of fresh air that penetrates my habitual defensive barriers and opens up larger horizons. In D. H. Lawrence's novel *The Rainbow,* the young hero's whole sense of life suddenly expands after his first significant sexual exchange with a woman, and he knows he will never be the same again. In contemplating this, he expresses a quality of wonder that most of us can probably recognize from our own experience:

> What was it all? There was a life so different from what he knew it. What was there outside his knowledge, how much? What was this that he had touched? What was he in this new influence? What did everything mean? Where was life, in that which he knew or all outside him?

Deeply connecting with another draws us out of ourselves. Our boundaries start to lose their familiar definition. Melting into the warmth of my beloved's arms, where do I leave off and where does she begin?

EARTHLY GROUNDEDNESS AND LIMITATION

If we focus only on feelings of heavenly expansion, however, we can easily get carried away and lose our center of gravity. We may become so merged with our partner that we lose track of our real needs and feelings, and this will eventually undermine even the most genuine loving connection. Or we may idealize love, seeing it as a stairway to the stars that provides an escape from earthly limitations: "Love is so fantastic! I feel so high! Let's get married, won't everything be wonderful!" Of course these expansive feelings are wonderful. But the potential distortion here is to imagine love as a blissful union that will save us from facing ourselves, the basic ache of our aloneness, our pain, and, ultimately, our death. Becoming too attached to the heavenly side of love leads to rude shocks and disappointments when we inevitably return to earth and have to deal with the real-life challenges of *making a relationship work.*

While the "high" of falling in love provides a taste of heavenly expansion, the earthly demands of two different individuals working out a day-to-day life together are what ground love and help it take root. When we try to make love all inspiration, it becomes shallow and inconsequential. Great love—the kind that illumines and transforms us—always includes a keen awareness of limitation as well. Though love may inspire us to expand and develop in new ways, we can never be all things to the one we love, or someone other than who we are. Yet once accepted, limitation also helps us develop essential qualities, such as patience, determination, compassion, and humor. When love comes down to earth—bringing to light those dark corners we would prefer to ignore, encompassing all the different parts of who we are—it gains depth and power.

INCLUDING BOTH SIDES OF OUR NATURE

Yet if neglecting earth is like having our head in the clouds, neglecting heaven is like slogging through the mud. For example, if we refuse to let go and expand our boundaries out of a need for control and security, we lose a sense of greater vision or adventure. Our relationship may become a kind of business deal, where everything must be negotiated. ("This is mine, that is yours," "I'll do this for you if you do that for me.") Or if we collude to play everything safe, it may become totally monotonous. Once we have lost a larger vision, we may try to fill the void that remains by creating a cozy materialistic lifestyle—watching television, acquiring upscale possessions, or climbing the social ladder.

Eventually, however, a life devoted to everyday routines and security concerns becomes too stale and predictable to satisfy the deepest longings of the heart. Playing out their habitual patterns and digging themselves deeper into their karma, a couple may fall asleep entirely. After twenty years of marriage, one of them may wake up, wondering "What have I done with my life?" and suddenly disappear in search of what has been lost.

Thus trying to make relationship a continual source of either bliss or security—all heaven or all earth—leaves us without a path. In holding on to pleasure, we try to keep ourselves *up*, refusing to come down to earth. Holding on to security keeps us *down*, so that we never venture to reach up at all.

Bringing the two sides of our nature together is an ongoing creative endeavor that continually takes us in new directions. If we neglect either the heights or the depths of our experience in our relationships, we can only stagnate. Only when we welcome both heaven and earth into a relationship—expanding our horizons, joining with our partner, and developing larger vision while also honoring our differences as individuals and attending to the practical details of everyday life—can our love gather power and momentum.

JOINING HEAVEN AND EARTH AWAKENS THE HEART

This is easy to say, but in practice quite difficult to do. Moving back and forth between togetherness and separateness, inspiration and practicality, is rarely smooth and easy. Indeed, the transition between these two states is often jarring and painful. Yet it is important to let ourselves feel this particular tension. In connecting us with the basic rawness at the core of our nature, it reminds us of what it means to be human. Thus all the rough edges we encounter in trying to bring together the opposites—freedom and commitment, vision and groundedness, letting go and taking hold, romance and reality, individuality and communion—are ways in which we forge our humanity and awaken our heart.

According to the ancient Chinese view, the genuine human being—one whose heart is awake to reality—is born in this intersection of heaven and earth. The upright human posture literally portrays the truth of this. Standing on the earth and raising our head upward exposes our heart to the world. Four-legged animals carefully protect the vulnerable soft front of the body. But as human beings we walk around with our heart exposed, allowing the world and other people to enter, touch, and move us. Only in this tenderness and openness to the whole of reality do we start to become fully human. Only in exposing the heart do we find a path.

4

Conditional and Unconditional Love

I falter before the task of finding the language to
express the incalculable paradoxes of love. Here is
the greatest and the smallest, the remotest and
nearest, the highest and lowest, and we cannot
discuss one side of it without also discussing the
other. Whatever one can say, no words express the
whole.

C. G. JUNG

WHENEVER OUR HEART OPENS to another person, we experience
a moment of unconditional love. People commonly imagine that
unconditional love is a high or distant ideal, one that is difficult,
if not impossible, to realize. Yet though it may be hard to put
into everyday practice, its nature is quite simple and ordinary:
opening and responding to another person's being without reservation.

We often glimpse this quality of love most vividly in begin-
nings and endings—at birth, at death, or when first falling in
love—when we are least under the influence of conditioned,
habitual patterns of perception. At such times, something vast
inside us connects with something vast in another. The other
person's sheer existence awakens us to the ordinary magic of
life. When our child is born, we do not have to decide to love
this infant—the feeling is choiceless, and flows forth freely.

When someone close to us is dying, we feel touched and present in an all-pervasive way that goes beyond all the little pros and cons of our relationship.

This unconditional quality of love arises from that which is unconditioned in us and responds to that which is unconditioned in another—the heart, that is, *our basic openness to reality.* This openness of the heart, which is born tender, responsive, and eager to reach out and touch the larger life around us, is not something we have to manufacture. It simply *is.*

It is the heart's desire to circulate human warmth freely back and forth, without putting limits or conditions on that exchange. When we love in this way, it alters our perceptions— everything in our world seems more colorful, vivid, and penetrating. When we are loved in this way, we feel acknowledged, seen, nourished, held. Moments of unconditional love allow us to touch the vastness and depth of human experience altogether.

And yet, as we know, this is not all there is to love. Because we are not just pure heart, but also live in an earthly form, we bring to relationships a collection of conditioned likes and dislikes, personal needs, cautions, and concerns that influence how deeply we can become involved with a particular person. When someone fits our personal needs and preferences, we feel pleasure and liking. This kind of attraction—which we could call conditional love—is a lesser form of love, in that it can fade away if the other person no longer continues to meet our needs.

CONFUSING THE TWO ORDERS OF LOVE

Relationships always contain both kinds of loving. Attraction to another person is usually most intense, and everything proceeds most smoothly, when they are in accord: The one we feel attracted to not only touches our heart, but also fits our personal conditions. Yet when these two orders of love do not mesh, it can be quite confusing. Someone may meet our conditions, yet somehow not move us very deeply. Or else someone may touch our heart, so that we want to say yes, while our personal criteria and considerations may lead us to say no. At the same time, our heart may look right past those things that jar our personal sensibilities, and rejoice in another person's very existence, despite all our reasonable intentions to maintain distance or play it safe. For in its deepest essence the heart knows nothing of conditions and is quite unreasonable. How then to proceed?

One common confusion at this point is to impose our conditional no on the yes of the heart: "I can only let myself feel this open *if* . . . she meets my needs . . . he loves me as much as I love him . . . she doesn't hurt me . . ." Yet our heart, whose nature is to say yes, only suffers when we try to constrict its openness by placing conditions on it. Although we may have to end or change the form of a relationship that does not meet our needs, we do not have to close down our heart. Trying to kill off the love that still wants to flow toward another human being constricts the very source of joy and aliveness inside us.

Another common confusion is to try to impose the yes of the heart on the no of our personal considerations. People often think that unconditional love means setting aside all their conditions and going along with whatever the person they love does. However, imagining that we should tolerate unconditionally anything our partner does can have devastating consequences. Unconditional love does not mean having to like something we in fact dislike or saying yes when we need to say no. Unconditional love arises from an entirely different place in us than conditional like and dislike, attraction and aversion. It is a being-to-being acknowledgment. And it responds to that which is unconditioned—the intrinsic goodness of another's open heart, beyond everything we may like or dislike about him or her. It is saying yes to another's being, but it does not mean always saying yes to *how* they are or *what* they do.

So just because our heart is open does not mean we must set aside all caution. Nor does setting conditions about what we want from a relationship have to negate the genuine openness we feel. Because relationships bring together heaven and earth, they always involve connecting from our deeper being *and* from our conditioned personality. While part of us might like to invite another person into our heart without reservation, another part of us wants to avoid being hurt, trapped, or abandoned. This is not a problem unless we become caught in a struggle between these two sides, feeling torn between unconditional love and our personal considerations. How then can we include both these sides of us in a relationship?

LOVE AND FEAR

Consider the kind of situation we find ourselves in when we are suddenly drawn to a new lover with tremendous force and intensity. This can be so exhilarating that we want to open without reservation. Yet at the same time we come up against inner cautions about letting our love flow so freely: "Can I let myself be this open? Will I lose myself or be swept away? Can I trust this person? Will she meet my needs? If so, will I become too dependent on her? Can I live with what I don't like about her? Can she accept me as I am and really be there for me? If not, could I be too badly hurt?"

If we listen to our heart, we may feel no reservations at all about becoming involved with this person. Yet as soon as we begin to consider what kind of relationship we want, we find ourselves in the realm of conditions. Feeling pulled in opposite directions—wanting to give ourselves freely while also honoring our considerations—may leave us uncertain about how to proceed.

At first we may imagine that this uncertainty is a sign that something is wrong. Yet it is natural to feel these opposite pulls. After all, we probably *have* been hurt before, so it is intelligent to exercise some caution this time. If we simply let our passion override our caution, we could be asking for trouble. But if we just let our fear close down our heart, we will never find out what a new relationship has to offer. Since there are no insurance policies in these matters, love, or risking the heart, and fear, or safeguarding the heart, arise together as intimate companions.

Here in the co-emergence of love and fear we feel the paradox of being human in a most poignant way. It would be so much easier if we could just remain self-contained and establish an impeccable set of conditions to protect us from risk. Or if we could simply open to someone without question, let ourselves go, and completely lose ourselves in merging together. Yet both these alternatives undermine love, *for they destroy the tension between self and other, known and unknown, that love actually thrives on.*

The key to finding our way in such situations lies in learning to allow opposite sides of our nature—unconditional and conditional love, passion and fear—to coexist, side by side, without letting one negate the other. When we do this, we become more fully present to our own experience and consequently to another person as well. We can let ourselves open and expand while still keeping our feet on the ground. In becoming more aware of the dynamic play and tension between the two sides of our nature, we begin to bring the whole of ourselves into a relationship.

Thus, some of the most powerful and penetrating moments in a relationship are those that bring us to an edge—where heaven and earth begin to connect with each other inside us. Here is where love leads into unknown territory and brings us most fully alive.

5

Dancing on the Razor's Edge

> When you live in tension, that is the best possible
> atmosphere for high creativity. That's where the
> void is and that's where God is: in between. We
> need a two-eyed view. Otherwise there will be no
> charge, no electricity; there will be no joy.
>
> FATHER WILLIAM McNAMARA

THE GREAT PARADOX OF LOVE is that it calls on us to be fully
ourselves and honor our individual truth (the earth principle),
while also letting go of self-centeredness, and giving without
holding back (the heaven principle). If we go too far out of
ourselves toward our partner, we start to lose ourselves, yet if
we hold back and remain too self-contained, no deep contact is
possible. If a relationship is to keep moving, we cannot get stuck
in any one-sided position. From moment to moment, we must
be able to stand our ground, yet also be able to let go and shift
our perspective when the situation changes (often the very next
moment!). We cannot cling to any secure, habitual stance—
either separateness or togetherness, dependence or independence, attachment or detachment.

Thus being genuinely present and intimate with another
person forces us to live on the edge of the unknown. Here we
are also on our growing edge, where old, familiar ways of being
leave off and new possibilities keep opening up before us. As

Paul Tillich put it, "the boundary is the best place for acquiring knowledge."

As the meeting point of two different worlds, a boundary or edge is a place of tremendous power. At the shore where sea and land meet, powerful, turbulent energies are released. Our skin is electric because it is where inside and outside, feeling and world, come together. Birth, marriage, and death are momentous passages because they transport us from one world to another. As the meeting point of light and dark, sunrise and sunset are the most vivid, poignant times of day. Similarly, as the joining of two different lives, intimate relationship stirs up tremendous energy, confusion, and creativity.

Since the essence of relationship is to bring opposites together, it continually provides opportunities to move between different parts of ourselves—male and female, known and unknown, love and fear, conditioned and unconditioned, heaven and earth. Love's alchemy thrives on this play, for it is the heat and friction of two people's differences that propel them to explore new ways of being. However, our fear of the unknown often tempts us to shut down and back away from the vibrant edge where opposites meet and sometimes clash. So, if we are to make use of the great opportunities that relationships present, we need to learn how to remain alert and open in face of the fear, tension, and ambiguity they arouse.

THE MEETING OF SELF AND OTHER IS
A RAZOR'S EDGE

The boundary where opposites meet is sharp, like a *razor's edge* because it cuts through the cozy, familiar set of habits and routines we identify as "me," "the way I am." We come upon this raw edge whenever we feel the sharpness of contact, the poignancy of being touched, affected, pierced by an *other*. As it says in the Upanishads, "Wherever there is other, there is fear." In opening to an *other*, we encounter the unknown; we feel vulnerable, uncertain what to do next. Open ourselves? Protect our-

selves? A little of each? What will become of us if we don't cling
to our old strategies? Where will this lead? These questions do
not go away, no matter how long we have been involved with
someone.

Indeed, the more we love and choose to commit ourselves
to another person, the more we can sense a potential devasta-
tion that could follow from this. We know that we must eventually lose this person, if only at the moment of death. What to do?
Protect ourselves by not loving so much? Leave and live in
isolation? Adopt a stoic philosophy? Our mind spins. None of
these are genuine or satisfying answers. They only distract us
from this razor's edge where we feel so sharply pierced by our
love and by our vulnerability about where it may lead. Yet we
need to feel pierced in this way. It brings us more fully awake
and alive.

Here on the razor's edge we discover the essential shaki-
ness of love's great balancing act. Yet here is where we can also
learn to dance with the flux and uncertainty continually occur-
ring in relationships. An acrobat does not maintain his poise on
a tightrope by trying to hold on to perfect balance. Instead, by
letting his balance shift back and forth, he keeps finding new
equilibrium. Similarly, an alive relationship is continually going
in and out of balance, rather than remaining in static harmony—
what D. H. Lawrence called a "stagnant unity." Opening to
another inevitably challenges our inner equilibrium as well, stirring up parts of ourselves that we have long been out of touch
with. *Thus each moment of uncertainty in a relationship indicates different
sides of ourselves or each other trying to come into new balance.* We can
only discover how to proceed in these moments by daring to feel
and acknowledge both sides, and seeing where that leads.

So instead of trying to hold on to some ideal state of harmony, we can learn to use the very act of starting to fall into one
extreme or the other to wake up and see where we are, and in
waking up, to find a new equilibrium. For instance, if my partner
and I start to feel disconnected—and this spurs us to explore
and talk about what is happening betwen us—this can help us
connect again, often in a new and richer way.

Of course, balancing on the razor's edge—exploring what it is like to be present with another person without relying on old formulas or strategies—can be quite scary. In this case, our fear is a reminder that we are moving from the familiar territory of our known ways into a larger unknown that lies ahead and all around. It warns us not to take anything for granted, to stay awake to what is happening and to what the situation calls for. The fear and rawness we feel when we have nothing solid to hold on to indicate that we are on our growing edge. So, though some have said that "love is letting go of fear," that view seems too simplistic. Since fear is the companion of intimacy, we could say instead that "love is making friends with fear."

CREATIVE TENSION

Feeling the pull of different tendencies inside us always produces a certain tension, which is uncomfortable at first. Yet this tension is a creative one, akin to what artists and other creative people feel before giving birth to a new work. In the art of Zen archery, the most important thing to learn is how to stand with bow fully drawn and release the arrow spontaneously at the point of maximum tension, without any deliberate effort. This is much more difficult than it sounds—it took one German student, Eugen Herrigel, four years of steady practice to learn. His teacher likened this process to snow falling off a bamboo leaf. The leaf keeps bending lower under the weight of the snow until the snow suddenly slips to the ground by itself, without the leaf having exerted any pressure.

Similarly, intimate relationships continually lead to moments of crisis and tension, which we cannot immediately see how to resolve. If we try to release the tension prematurely, this is like *trying* to shoot the arrow—we will likely miss the genuine resolution that could really lead us forward. Resting awhile at the point of maximum tension, feeling and trusting the rawness that arises there, is what I mean by balancing on the razor's edge. If we wait there alertly, the leaf will bend low enough for the snow to fall off by itself, and the way forward can become clear.

Once when the Buddha was asked about the optimal way to be, he answered, using the analogy of a stringed instrument, "Not too tight and not too loose." Even the Buddha could not define or formulate this state; he could only say what it was *not*, and invite his questioner to find it for himself. Likewise, we learn to flow with the shifting dance of self and other only through trial and error—now becoming too stiff and controlled, now losing our footing and tripping over ourselves—until we begin to find our own natural balance point.

When falling in love, we may at first try to resolve the tension and uncertainty we feel by pitting different sides of ourselves against each other and trying to force a decision: "Propose to her right now before you miss your chance!" Or "Run for your life before you get in any deeper." But since these alternatives are the product of our busy oppositional mind, which can grasp only one side of any polarity at a time, they lead nowhere. Such impossible choices only throw us into a state of ambivalence, which is very different from dynamically balancing on the razor's edge. Ambivalence is a vacillating attempt to choose sides—now one, now the other—instead of letting both sides stay active until we find an equilibrium.

We can learn to balance on the razor's edge only by staying present with our sense of uncertainty, rather than taking sides in our inner debate. When we give up preconceived agendas about what *should* happen and open to the energy in our uncertainty instead, we become more present and discerning. Then we may see how our fear is trying to argue us out of our love, or how our passion is trying to override our caution. Only through boycotting this struggle—neither suppressing nor indulging either side—can we begin to dance on the razor's edge.

When we take our seat and face into our fear, without either fighting against it or letting it take us over, we also draw on a deeper resource within us: our warrior spirit. And this is of far greater benefit than trying to make ourselves feel comfortable by getting rid of our fear.

When we look at our fear in this way, we can also begin to see some humor in the situation. Suppressing fears makes them deadly serious, whereas exposing them—perhaps even naming all our catastrophic expectations until we see their absurdity—can help us take them more lightly and even play with them. Humor, which often arises out of nowhere when everything otherwise seems bleak or impossible, is one creative way of dancing with the tension of opposites. In moments of humor, the snow falls from the leaf, so to speak—the mind suddenly expands, allowing us to relax with incongruity. Contradiction and ambiguity no longer require a struggle, and we can begin to soften.

Bravery, discernment, humor, and gentleness—these are but a few of the qualities we discover when we let ourselves balance on the razor's edge, instead of jumping to premature conclusions. Opening to the whole of what is happening—our love *and* our fear—forces us to stretch to include very different parts of ourselves. And this is how we grow—through integrating seemingly dissonant, incompatible elements into a larger whole. Only then can we give up struggling and find our way forward by letting the situation unfold at its own pace. In this way, balancing on the razor's edge reveals a path.

A doctor I once worked with whose wife was on the verge of leaving him kept desperately trying to make things right so that he would not lose her. Yet nothing seemed to do any good, for his wife could tell that Gregory cared more about keeping her from leaving than with connecting in a new and deeper way. He was trying to control the situation, and his perpetual need to be in control was one of her greatest grievances against him. When Gregory realized this, he veered to the other extreme: venting his pain and anguish in uncontrolled outbursts. Yet this was not a real letting go; it was just another strategy to influence his wife. Gregory had always believed that he should know what to do in every situation. Now he had finally encountered a situation where every attempt to find the right solution only made things worse.

Ironically, trying so hard to find "the right way to be" kept

Gregory from being genuinely present. It was not until he became so exasperated that he gave up hope of "fixing" the marriage that he found, almost by accident, a new way to be with the situation. When he gave up trying to win over his wife and simply opened instead to his own experience, something inside him suddenly lit up. He was back in touch with his own spirit, which made him softer and more real. He also displayed a gallows humor that was quite appealing. The snow had slipped from the leaf! Of course, as soon as his wife responded favorably to this new way of being, he became hopeful about winning her back again and reverted to his old habits. Only by returning to the razor's edge—staying open to his experience from moment to moment, instead of trying to make things better—could he be present to himself and thus contact his wife in a way she could respond to.

LEANING INTO THE EDGE

Oddly enough, this spot where we come most alive in a relationship is often, at first glance, where we would least like to be. We would rather jump to a conclusion than open to our uncertainty. Or, like Gregory, we want to fix things, not give up struggling so hard for solutions. Similarly, two partners who are fighting often want to put an end to their conflict without ever opening to how it actually touches them. Yet no matter how difficult a relationship conflict is, we can always find a way forward by leaning into the sharp, vibrant edge it puts us in touch with.

A few minutes after my partner and I have had a big argument and withdrawn to different parts of the house, we pass each other in the hall and pause, looking tentatively in each other's eyes. Part of me just wants to drop my grievances and reach out to her. It says to me, "Stop being so caught in your emotions. Life is short. Put aside your grievance and take her in your arms." At the same time, another part of me wants to argue my side further and let her know just how angry I am. This part says, "The issue we're arguing about is important. How can I feel loving when I'm so angry with her about this? She will think I'm a pushover and that she can walk all over me.''

For a moment, I feel uncertain, not knowing which way to turn. If I suppress my anger, that only cuts me off from my feelings and makes me less present. Yet if I just hold on to my anger, it becomes a rigid stance that keeps us apart. Both these sides belong to me, yet neither speaks for all of me. If I struggle to resolve these opposing points of view, I remain at an impasse. Only by accepting all that I feel at this moment—"I'm angry at you *and* I still love you"—do I come back to the sharp edge of the present moment.

Recognizing these different parts of me without leaping to one "solution" or another leaves me feeling somewhat raw and shaky. Yet if I can stay on this edge where I don't know what to do, without falling back into some old pattern—such as blaming her, justifying myself, or denying my anger—then for a moment my awareness flirts with new possibilities. This sharp edge keeps jogging me loose from holding on to any position: Here we both are, feeling raw with each other, not knowing what to do next.

Feeling all this is bittersweet. It is sad and a little funny to contain such different impulses, to want to yell at her one moment and hold her in my arms the next. Staying present with the poignancy of this, leaning into it instead of resisting it, I suddenly sense something shifting inside. We start to make contact at a level below the conflict, and as this happens, the stalemate between us naturally starts to loosen. *In our rawness we connect more deeply.* An unreasonable spark of warmth starts to kindle in me. I am feeling my love once more, without conditions, not because she is how I want her to be, but because we are fully there with each other again. This provides inspiration to relate to our conflict in a new way.

Standing there in the hallway, as we open to the whole of our experience, we soften, and can start to listen to each other again. The tension between us gives way to humor. We playfully call each other names, expressing our anger and our affection at the same time. As we talk about our feelings and concerns, we are more open to hearing each other's point of view. Because we are connecting with each other from our rawness, instead of from entrenched positions, we can discuss the cause of our conflict more openly, without making each other defensive. By bringing to light aspects of our life together that need our attention, this incident leads somewhere. It becomes a step on our path.

In this way, through acknowledging the rough edges of our humanness, we *learn more deeply how to love.* Love in the fullest, richest sense is not just something that falls in our lap like manna from heaven, but something that we must learn. Granted, the first flush of love, the spontaneous arising of unconditional openness, just happens, without any work or effort on our part. Yet as our fears and conditions enter the picture, and difficult parts of a relationship begin to emerge, our love is put to the test. Through feeling the painful discrepancy between the boundless love in our heart and the limited ways it manifests, we are moved to bring that love more fully into our lives. Love in this more developed sense involves learning to embrace the whole of our experience, including everything that we find most difficult to accept.

By teaching us to include all of ourselves—courage and fear, celebration and pain, expansiveness and limitation—love helps us become both tough and tender at the same time. This strength that is also soft and gentle is the true child of the union of man and woman. Every couple struggling to learn to love partakes in the labor of this birth.

PART II

Personal Path

Threading its way along the boundary between our larger being and our karmic patterns, joining heaven and earth, the path of love has both a personal and a sacred side. On the personal level, intimate relationship calls on us to expand our capacities and develop greater wholeness as individuals. Beyond that, the love between man and woman also presents a sacred challenge: to go beyond the single-minded pursuit of purely personal gratifications and tap into the larger energies of life as a whole. When love becomes a vehicle for tuning in to the great mysteries of creation all around us, it provides a deeper sense of purpose and direction. The personal and the sacred are two overlapping sides of one and the same path.

6

Falling in Love:
Passion as Path

Without warning,
As a whirlwind swoops upon an oak,
Love shakes my heart.

SAPPHO

Great love can both take hold and let go.

A. R. ORAGE

SUDDENLY, OUT OF NOWHERE, we are struck by the expression on another's face, how he or she speaks, moves, or looks at us. Some quality of beauty penetrates us and almost makes us ache, stirring a desire to reach out and make contact. This is the energy of passion.

Love's passion is a powerful force that has both inspired and destroyed countless lovers through the ages. One moment it can feel like divine grace; the next moment it can sweep us away in a torrent of hopes and fears that blind us, bend us out of shape, and leave us hurt and disillusioned. As a student of mine once remarked, "No experience has ever made me feel so intensely alive, yet so confused and out of touch at the same time." We have no idea where this intensity of feeling comes from, why it drives us as it does, or where it will lead. No wonder so many people are either addicted to falling in love or scared to death of it, or both at the same time.

In societies where arranged marriages are the norm, falling in love is rare and of little consequence. When it does appear, it is dismissed as a temporary form of madness, a youthful folly. In our society, we accord it greater importance, since it gives birth to the romantic feelings that often lead to marriage. Yet its sudden eruption has also torn many marriages and lives apart. So our culture is tremendously ambivalent toward passion, alternately glorifying it as a stairway to heaven—that will lift us above the pain of the world—and denouncing it as a pathway to hell—that will drag us down into the mire of animal lust. Some writers regard falling in love as a rare moment of clearly perceiving another person's deepest essence. Others see it as a hormonal frenzy, or in Scott Peck's words, "a trick our genes pull on [us] to hoodwink us into marriage."

How can falling in love stir up such different reactions and lead to such opposite conclusions? Must passion inevitably breed illusion, causing us to lose our seat and act in ways we later regret? Or can it help us bridge the two sides of our nature and thus connect with life more wholeheartedly? Can a couple continue to draw on it for energy and inspiration, even after many years of being together? Since passion provides powerful fuel propelling a couple's journey forward, it is important to distinguish what is real in this experience from what is delusional. Relating to passion in a sane and healthy way is the first and one of the greatest challenges in a relationship.

THE SPARK OF PASSION

Passion is the spark of excitement we feel when we stand on the edge of the unknown. It arises at the boundary where two different worlds rub up against each other—male and female, self and other, inner and outer, familiar patterns and uncharted possibilities. As D. H. Lawrence put it, "What is the beloved? She is that which I am not." In one of his poems Lawrence conveys this impassioned sense of wonder:

I put out my hand in the night, one night, and my
  hand
touched that which was verily not me . . .
it was the unknown . . .
The other, she has strange green eyes!
And land that beats with a pulse!
Also she . . . has strange-mounded breasts and
strange sheer slopes, and white levels . . .
I touched her flank and knew I was carried . . .
over to the new world . . .

When we fall in love, a new world opens up. Leaping across
the boundary of self and other, the spark of passion "lights up
the night," providing sudden glimpses of mystery and depth.
Passion is an intense quality of *energized presence* that puts us in
touch with the fullness and richness of being alive.

We can fall in love in little ways at any moment. Suddenly
something or someone takes our breath away. We feel an expansive or fluttery sensation in our chest. And we taste what it is like
to be fully present, if only for a fleeting instant. This can happen
upon waking to a fine spring morning, with the sunlight filtering
through the new greenery, upon suddenly catching a glimpse of
the open sea after long traveling, or when the ripe, pungent
earth fills our senses on a crisp autumn afternoon. I have found,
at times of heightened perception, such as on meditation re-
treats or in groups of people who are communicating deeply,
that it is not hard to fall in love several times a day; that is, to
keep finding myself deeply moved not only by the people there,
but also by the landscape, the sounds of the forest, the moon at
night, or the changing patterns of wind, light, clouds, and rain.
Although this vividness of perception may seem special, it is also
quite ordinary. If it be magic, it is ordinary magic, because it is
only a keener awareness of what is already there. Though we
cannot hold on to such moments, they leave us with a sense of
what life could be like if we could live more often at this threshold of vivid presence.

PASSION: CONDITIONAL AND UNCONDITIONAL

Passion's essential nature is spontaneous and unconditional because it is unfabricated. Since our very being is open to begin with, it naturally resonates and wants to connect with what is greater than ourselves—the vastness of life itself. Passion is the feeling of life wanting to connect with life; life inside us connecting with life outside.[1] To fall in love is to feel the basic openness of our being.

The swelling of passion, which makes us feel so full and rich, makes our usual state of distraction and disconnectedness seem pale and impoverished by contrast. Yet here is where we also start to fall into delusion, for we usually imagine the object of our passion to be the source of this newfound fullness. This makes us try to grasp and hold on to the one who sparks such an intense feeling of aliveness inside us.

The inexhaustible richness of life is, in Buddhist terms, a "wish-fulfilling gem" because it provides us with everything we need. Yet when we fall in love, we usually imagine the beloved, rather than life itself, to be the wish-fulfilling gem who could make all our dreams come true. So, to the extent that we do not feel deeply connected with the life moving inside us, we come to depend on something outside ourselves to enrich us.

In regarding the focus of our passion—the beloved—as a treasure to possess, we convert our unconditional passion into something conditional and grasping: "How alive I would feel, how beautiful life would be, *if only* this person belonged to me." Yet grasping at another person only magnifies our inner sense of poverty and leads to the torments of romantic addiction and obsession. Love becomes a drug, and the loved one becomes the addicted lover's "fix."[2]

Unconditional passion has no agenda. It is like the freely radiating energy of the sun. Yet if I identify my beloved as the source of this powerful energy, then *I must have her*—and my passion turns into an obsessive, blinding, fatal attraction. No wonder the great love tales usually end in tragedy. Those who try to carry such a burden for others, such as Romeo and Juliet, or even Marilyn Monroe, die young.

Yet it is important to distinguish here between seeing another as the *source* of our passion—which always leads to distortion and addiction—and allowing another to be the *focus* of our passion—which is not in itself a problem. Passion becomes problematic when we confuse *focus* with *source*, imagining that the one toward whom our passion flows is the *cause* of our feeling so alive. The natural activity of passion is to connect intensely—whether it be with the color of the sky, our life's work, or the presence of our beloved. Of course, we do not feel equally passionate toward just anyone or anything that comes along—only certain forms or qualities awaken our energy and inspire it to flow toward them. Yet when we imagine that the conditional focus of our passion is the unconditional source of our aliveness, we throw ourselves into a state of inner impoverishment and confusion. Peter Trachtenberg, in his book *The Casanova Complex*, describes this kind of tormented passion in this way:

> When I met a woman who attracted me, my desire for her was immediate and crippling—a hammer blow to the heart. In the beginning there was just that longing, and the sense of myself as a starving orphan gazing through a window at a happy family sitting down to dinner . . . I had to see her again and again, to conquer her in different ways. It might take a few days to a few years—a whole relationship based on hunger and frustration.

Yet he eventually understood that nothing outside him could fill his inner sense of poverty, for he concludes: "For my part, I yearned for something no woman could ever give me."

IDOLIZING THE BELOVED

What is it, then, that the lover really yearns for? Consider the situation of Joanna, a woman in her early thirties who had been driven to despair by a series of brief affairs that led nowhere. She would repeatedly find herself building up intense feelings about men after a few dates, based on wild, unrealistic dreams of total fulfillment. At first she would inflate a lover to epic proportions, only to crash in disillusion within a few weeks or months. Then she would go through a period of cynical isolation until the next potential savior came along. She came in for counseling out of a need to understand why her passion took such strange turns, firing her up with inflated hopes one moment and then just as suddenly dashing her on the ground. She no longer trusted that she could feel passionate without becoming swept away by tides of uncontrollable fantasies and emotions. How could such an otherwise intelligent and perceptive woman repeatedly endow her lovers with an almost godlike status? What was she really looking for?

Idolizing someone we fall in love with is an example of a strange trick we play on ourselves—what psychologists call *projection.* Simply stated, this means heightened sensitivity to certain qualities in another person that we fail to acknowledge in ourselves. The classic example is the person who does not acknowledge his own aggression, but imagines that other people are out to get him.

When romantically idolizing someone, we project not our own unacknowledged negative feelings, but all the power, beauty, and richness of our being, which we usually fail to recognize inside us. Human nature is vast. Our being actually reflects and contains the whole range of peaceful and wrathful energies of heaven and earth, fire and water, sun and stars. But we usually inhabit only a small portion of our being. We live on the island of our conditioned self, a complex of memories, notions, and images of ourselves that constitute our identity as we know it. Yet the larger expanse of our being—its vastness, intensity, and depths—we do not usually identify as intimately our own. Even though this larger being is more truly who we are—since it is not an invention, like our self-images—we do not know it as our true nature.

Since we have a hard time perceiving our own vastness and

beauty, we project it outward instead, where it is easier to see. Just as the individual who denies his anger finds it coming back at him from the world, so we discover the radiance of our own being in and through our beloved, who mirrors it back to us. We are dazzled by what we see. We want it, we must have it at any cost. Since we can't live without it—for it is, after all, our own being—we wind up not only addicted, but further alienated from ourselves as well.

Certainly this was true for Joanna. She felt fully alive only when she was in a relationship with a man. Most psychoanalysts would explain this as a result of her early childhood, when she tried to win the favors of her father, whom she saw as larger than life. Indeed, our choice of intimate partners is always partly determined by old images based on unfulfilled childhood wishes and needs. This template of images that we carry from the past is what produces the particular distortions—the typical kinds of unrealistic fantasies and conflicting emotions—that we each go through when we fall in love.

Nonetheless, something larger still wants to shine through this overlay from the past. How could we envision such radiance and beauty in others in the first place if we did not already have some sense of power and greatness inside us? At the root of Joanna's need to win her father's love was a deeper, more basic need to feel the goodness and fullness of her own being, and to know that it was indeed worth celebrating.

Abraham Maslow once wrote that "we are generally afraid to become that which we glimpse in our most perfect moments," no doubt because our larger being threatens us in many ways. If we were to open to it fully, perhaps it would disrupt our cozy little habits and throw our familiar, small identity into question. So, just as early peoples worshiped as gods what they feared and did not understand, so we, who are primitives in regard to our larger being, tend to worship our greater powers at a safe distance, by letting others carry them for us. Thus we "fall" for the beloved, whom we place above us, granting him or her power to uplift us from our "fallen" state of hunger and unworthiness.

Idolizing the beloved inflates us and makes us feel "high," as the lofty metaphors used to describe this state suggest.

PASSION AND DEVOTION

In this way, our unconditional passion, which is a genuine long-ing to connect with the vastness of life, gets converted into an addictive obsession. Yet the belief that our wealth of feeling comes from the object of our passion, whom we must therefore possess, is not just a personal delusion. It is also widely pro-moted by our culture at large and is a common theme in count-less plays, movies, books, and love songs. How many songs on the radio do we hear that are variations on the theme of "You are everything, I am nothing"? ("You're the better part of me," "You are my only sunshine," "I can't live, if living is without you," "I've got to have you, baby," etc.) Yet if this were just a Hollywood fabrication, it would not have such a deep hold at every level of our society. What makes it such a powerful cultural theme is that it represents a convergence of psychological, spiri-tual, and historical factors—which together create a web of illu-sion from which it is hard to extricate ourselves.

The fantasy that our beloved can save us is the distorted form of a powerful idea from the courtly love tradition, from which all our notions of romantic love derive. The troubadour poetry of twelfth-century France taught that the romantic feel-ing between man and woman was a vehicle for connecting with the divine. The deep human urge to connect with something greater than ourselves—which had been the exclusive province of religion—now took a secular form. The troubadour songs were influenced by the poetry of Sufism, the mystical branch of Islam, which expressed intense devotional longing for the divine or the spiritual master, addressed as "the Beloved." The trouba-dour imported this fervent devotional sentiment into his poetry, directing it toward his Lady, rather than to God.

Yet although courtly love took place between man and woman, rather than between humanity and God, it still retained a spiritual orientation. In its purest form, a knight would fall in love with a woman who was already married, but would forego sexual consummation with her. This was an ingenious device that allowed a lover to use the power of his passion for his own transformation.[3] With sexual conquest ruled out, the trials he had to undergo in the service of his lady became a path of character development and spiritual purification. The refining quality of such a love helped him develop new sensitivities and realize that era's new ideal—to become a "gentle man."

By falling in love with someone he could not expect to attain, the courtly lover could experience the two sides of passion simultaneously. While focusing his desire on the finite form of his Lady (conditional passion), he also had to let go of possessing her, which threw him back into the pure intensity of his feeling, to the source of unconditional passion inside himself. This combination of intensely focusing his passion, while having to let go of grasping, put him on the razor's edge, and this allowed him to open up in new ways.

When we sit on the razor's edge, *consciously* directing our love toward an object we know we can never possess, passion can ripen into something deeper—devotion. Wholehearted devotion, whether it be to a loved one, a spiritual master, or ultimate truth, is a powerful, transformative energy that can work magic on the human soul. Recognizing this, many religious traditions have developed devotional practices that harness this energy for spiritual purposes.[4] Since the devotee cannot possess the object of devotion—God or the spiritual master—devotional practice requires him to relinquish fixation, so that he may discover the fullness of his love as *the treasure of his own heart.* This awakens him from the poverty of depending on others to the richness of his deeper being, which he can then begin to share more fully with others.

The romantic devotional practice of courtly love was so powerful that it still shapes how we fall in love eight hundred years later.[5] Yet we have lost touch with the original transformative purpose of this practice. Although our romantic ideas still echo the sentiments of the troubadours, we differ from them in expecting a real-life relationship to fill what is essentially a spiritual longing. Lacking any sense of how passion could be a devotional path for tapping greater powers inside us, we imagine that we can find some kind of salvation through taking possession of an ideal "golden princess" or "knight in shining armor." So instead of being purified by love, we often wind up reduced to a state of addiction or dependency, feeling bitter when we fail to find our hoped-for salvation. Passion becomes a torment, and our devotional feelings become enslaving rather than liberating. In the words of the Sufi master, Hazrat Inayat Khan:

> The sorrow of the lover is continual, in the presence and absence of the beloved: in the presence for fear of the absence, and in absence in longing for the presence. The pain of love becomes in time the life of the lover.

ROMANTIC AGONY

The longing to devote ourselves to something we regard as greater than ourselves is a beautiful quality. But when we fail to recognize its essential nature—as a basic need to realize the fullness of our larger being—falling in love can leave us feeling helpless and tortured, like Joanna in her obsessions with men. Here we see the relation between the words *passion* and *passive*. In falling under the spell of her lovers, Joanna saw herself as a passive victim—a state of mind commonly portrayed in the classic love tales. Tristan feels driven toward Isolde not out of choice, but because he has accidentally swallowed a love potion. In the most famous of Sufi love tales, Majnun laments that his passion for Layla, which causes him to go mad and wander the countryside composing love songs, is completely beyond his control: "I have not chosen the way, I have been cast upon it. I am manacled, and my fetters are made of iron. But it was not I who forged them; it was my Kismet that decided. I follow obediently my beloved, who owns my soul."

Eventually this agony itself may become addicting, because

its burning intensity makes us feel so alive. Thus is born the classic romantic melodrama: The lover's struggle to overcome the obstacles between himself and his beloved keeps the fire of his passion burning at a feverish pitch. Yet while struggling to win his beloved, the lover also unconsciously sabotages any genuine relationship with her, so that he can maintain the vivid intensity of his longing. If he actually gets to know his beloved—as an ordinary, imperfect person, with the same sorts of needs and failings as himself—he will no longer be able to sustain the illusion that makes him feel so high.

Thus we often unconsciously choose partners who are unattainable, because of marriage, age, geographical distance, or emotional incompatibility. Or else we may start fights that create distance just when we are getting too close. This keeps us stuck in the neurotic runaround that is the stuff of all soap operas: seeking fulfillment and denying it to ourselves at the same time. As Majnun proclaims to Layla: "You are my salve for a hundred thousand wounds, yet you are also my sickness."

LOVE AND DEATH

Addictive passion is thus a no-win situation—in Majnun's words, a "riddle without a solution, a code which none can decipher." The only solution for Layla and Majnun is the classic denouement of countless tragic romances: death. Thus, paradoxically, passion, which starts out making us feel so intensely alive, brings us to a consideration of death.

What is the death of the lovers pointing to? As a symbol, it contains important clues about how we can overcome addictive passion, while still enjoying the larger unconditional passion at the root of the male/female connection.

At one level, the lovers' death suggests that addiction to anything we use to make ourselves feel high must eventually lead to destruction. The tale of Axel and Sara—a gem of nineteenth-century melancholy romanticism by Villiers de l'Isle-Adam—clearly illustrates this. Axel, a lonely, brooding young count, meets Sara in the treasury of his castle, where they instantly fall in love. After feasting on delicious fantasies about how they could run away together, using his riches to travel the world and taste its infinite delights, Axel decides that they should instead commit suicide at the height of their passion. He knows that everyday life could never measure up to the dreams that have set their hearts ablaze:

> To consent, after this, to live would be but sacrilege against ourselves. Live? Our servants will do that for us.

In choosing the heavenly illusion of addictive passion, they must sacrifice earthly reality. In Axel's words, "The quality of our hope no longer allows us the earth."

In everyday life, addiction to passion may lead to death in different sorts of ways. The jilted lover who kills his beloved because he "loves her so much" is one example. More commonly, couples who try to hold on to their passion by keeping it in a fixed mold often do real damage to their relationship. As one woman described the death that occurred in her marriage:

> I was afraid of losing my passion. I wanted to feel it on demand, even in the middle of my pregnancy when I was not naturally feeling sexual. I needed it to let me know that I was alive, and to prove that our relationship was still okay. When I didn't feel it, I blamed our relationship. By trying to hold on so hard to my passion, I killed it and the marriage too.

Yet the death that intervenes in the classic love tales also has a deeper significance. It points to the necessity of letting go, which, though it may seem like a death, can also take us beyond the snares and dead ends of romantic illusion. What must die, when we let the deeper current of our passion flow freely, is our small, impoverished view of ourselves and, along with that, our attempt to grasp on to another person to save us.

Some years ago I had a powerful realization about the connection between love and death. One day, during a meditation retreat in the Rocky Mountains, as my ideas about who I was began to fall away, I started to feel more vividly alive and present. Soon, however, this liberating feeling turned to fear. Out of this fear arose an elaborate fantasy about marrying the woman in my life. But then, just as the marriage ceremony ended and we were enjoying our new union, the thought struck like lightning: "What if she dies? What if I die?" Once again, nothing to hold on to. Suddenly, with a jolt, I found myself back in my cabin in the Rockies.

The next morning, waking up before dawn in a dreamlike state, I imagined I was dying. (I had been having trouble breathing at that altitude and felt constricted in my chest.) I considered how to prepare myself for death, but nothing felt quite right. Finally it became clear that all I could do was to let love flow freely through me, without trying to stay in control. As I felt what that was like, I found that I could give in to dying. The constriction in my chest began to ease, the sun was coming up, and I looked out of my sleeping bag to find another day beginning.

Reflecting on this, I saw the connection between my experiences of these two days. On the first day, when my sense of identity fell away and I had a glimpse of pure passionate presence to life, I had become afraid of that free egoless energy because it gave me nothing to hold on to. So I had converted my unconditional passion into a specific longing, directed toward the woman I imagined marrying. My fantasy had been an attempt to save myself from the little death I was experiencing as my identity dissolved. Yet it too led to the same place: "What if we die?" And so I had to face death, coming to terms with it only by letting my love for life run through my body without restraint. So, just as love makes death all the more poignant, death makes loving all the more essential. Dying requires us to love and let go; love requires us to die and let go.

PASSION AND SURRENDER

Thus if passion is a great stream of life energy surging through us, its natural course is to *lead to surrender,* like a river that must empty into the sea. Even in my very first moments of attraction to a woman, I can sense a surrender that must follow if I pursue her. In wanting to move toward her, I feel moved, in ways I cannot control. In wanting to reach out and touch her, I feel touched, in my most sensitive spots. If I open to my passion and let it move freely in me, it forces me to let go, give in, and feel how raw and vulnerable I truly am.

No wonder my first impulse may be to seduce her. When passion pierces me and resonates through every fiber of my being, grasping and seducing are ways of trying to regain control of the situation and not feel so disarmed. Yet the more I try to control my passion—either by engaging in conquests and melodramas or by suppressing it—the more *it* drives and controls *me.* Although I would like to possess the aliveness of passion without having to go through the death of surrendering, this is not possible. Passion and surrender are two halves of one whole cycle. The river must return to the sea that is its source so that its waters can keep on flowing.

The surrender that passion calls for involves letting go of holding on: to myself—my fascination with getting high or being saved—and to my partner—my attempt to grasp or control her. To let go in this way can feel like a death, for it means giving up old ways of trying to make myself feel alive or secure. Yet what is most alive in me *wants* these old ways to die, so that it can expand and move more freely. No wonder falling in love makes us rejoice and tremble at the same time: It calls us toward the death of our old self.

In one of his poems, Goethe calls our urge to die and be transformed a "holy longing," likening it to a moth, "insane for the light," drawn toward the flames of a candle:

> I praise what is truly alive,
> what longs to be burned to death.

And his conclusion is simple and unequivocal:

> And so long as you haven't experienced
> this: to die and so to grow,
> you are only a troubled guest
> on this dark earth.

Making love is the literal embodiment of passion turning into surrender. The whole unfolding of passion—from approach, to pursuit, to courtship, and all the rest—builds toward a moment of orgasmic letting go, in which we feel full and empty at the same time—full of life and empty of self. As we move toward orgasm we can't hold on to our partner, we can't hold on to life, we can't even hold on to our sexual excitement. We have to let it all go. Orgasm carries us across the threshold of the great unknown, beyond the mind, beyond pleasure, beyond the beloved, beyond even relationship itself. It is, as the French say, "the little death *(la petite mort)."*

So in following our passion all the way, we arrive at the boundary of life and death; here we feel the insignificance of our small self as we enter into the greater mystery from which we come and to which we must return. No wonder we cling so tightly to our passion: It is a way of fighting off the experience of death. Yet though we may try to hold on to it for dear life, passion's aim is much larger. As the agent of love's unquenchable thirst for wholeness, passion seeks to connect us with the whole of reality, with life and death altogether.

PASSION AS PATH

Because romantic passion has led to countless broken lives and marriages, many people have turned against it and condemned it altogether. Writers such as Denis de Rougemont, Scott Peck, and Robert Johnson regard it as the antithesis of mature human love. As de Rougemont writes, "Passion-love is . . . an impoverishment of one's being . . . *Passion wrecks the very notion of marriage."*

What these writers rightly criticize is the misguided attempt to make a relationship the main source of our spiritual fulfillment. Yet in trying to set things straight, they go to the other extreme—discounting any larger dimension of passion altogether. When Peck writes, "Love is not a feeling, [but] an act of will," he is arguing for all work, no play, for earth at the expense of heaven. In so doing, he fails to appreciate the unconditional nature of passion—as a deep resonance with life's great beauty—underneath all the distorted forms it may take. Devaluing passion or trying to exclude it from marriage only diminishes the vital spark between a man and a woman that propels their journey forward. This leaves us stuck with a hollow, stagnant form, along with an irresistible urge to break out of its constraints.

So while indulging in addictive passion promotes delusion and death, denouncing passion altogether only maintains the crippling schism between heaven and earth—romantic inspiration and marital commitment—that has plagued love in the Western world for centuries. Neither inflating passion nor condemning it gives us a path.

The heavenly side of passion is an ecstatic urge to break out of our habitual patterns and realize a vaster sense of being. Yet unless we can ground this energy, by bringing it into an I–Thou relationship, it will take a distorted form. When we split off its heavenly side from earth, we "fall in love with love," becoming more enamored with our own excitement than with the reality of an ongoing partnership. Fearing that bringing passion down to earth will ruin our high, we are unwilling to bring it into one-pointed focus, to engage with a real person with any constancy or commitment, to *take hold.*

At the other extreme, if we overemphasize passion's earthly side at the expense of heaven, we cannot *let go,* or relax our focus on a particular person, whom we *must have* and *cannot live without.* In the heavenly distortion, addiction to our own excitement prevents us from devoting ourselves to another person. In the earthly distortion, addiction to the other person prevents us from feeling the larger source of aliveness within ourselves.

When we can bring these two sides together, joining heaven and earth, true devotion—*passion without fixation*—becomes possible.

The key to overcoming the torments of passion lies in realizing that this energy arises from our larger being and can never be entirely satisfied by any finite person or thing. Its intrinsic nature is egoless and pure in that it is ultimately a desire to experience the fullness of life itself. Whether it leads to devotion and surrender or else to fixation and addiction *depends on what we do with it.*

For passion to become path, we must learn to dance on the razor's edge of this energy—now taking hold, now letting go, now focusing our passion with single-pointed intensity, now releasing its focus and feeling its source in the life flowing deep within us. In this way, we can begin to ride the energy of desire instead of getting swept away by it. We can let it resonate through us and flow toward others without having to cling to them.

As we learn to keep our seat and ride our passion, we also become more open to the little flashes of falling in love that are always available: with a leaf falling through the air, the red sun rising behind a range of darkened hills, or a face that we glimpse on the street. These flashes do not have to mean anything terribly serious—we surely don't have to chase after everything that stirs our passion. By simply appreciating the pure quality of this energy as it arises in the moment, we can let ourselves fall in love lightly, without becoming obsessed.

In an ongoing relationship, a couple's passion may express itself in many different ways. Sometimes it will roar like a mountain torrent. Sometimes it will lie still and contained, like a deep, quiet pool. And sometimes it will flow gently like a broad stream meandering across the plains, or carelessly like a river emptying into the sea. Changing like the weather and the seasons, a couple's passion could be romantic and sweet, sad and tender, or fierce and driving, depending on the circumstances. If they can let their passion move freely, it will keep finding new and different forms of expression—not just in making love, but also in cooking a meal, going for a walk, having a fight, or just sharing their thoughts and feelings. It will begin to suffuse every aspect of their relationship, becoming a magnetic bond that will hold them together through the most difficult of times.

When two people recognize the true nature of their passion—as a powerful, radiant heart energy that wants to shine forth, flow freely, and connect with life at large—they will not need to suppress this feeling or try to maintain a feverish intensity. This will keep their love fresh, and allow them to keep falling in love with the phenomenal world and with each other, again and again.

7

Breaking the Heart—Open

> Your heart is not living until it has experienced
> pain . . . The pain of love breaks open the heart,
> even if it is as hard as a rock.
>
> HAZRAT INAYAT KHAN

A RELATIONSHIP that has any depth and power at all will inevitably penetrate our usual shield of defenses, exposing our most tender and sensitive spots, and leaving us feeling vulnerable—literally, "able to be wounded." To love, in this sense, is to open ourselves to being hurt. The dream of love would have us believe that something is wrong if a relationship causes us pain. Yet trying to avoid the wound of love only creates a more permanent kind of damage. It prevents us from opening ourselves fully, and this keeps us from ever forming a deeply satisfying intimate connection.

Depending on how we relate to love's pain, it can lead in one of two very different directions. If we regard it as a threat, something to avoid at all cost, we will try to patch it over, keep it out of sight. After a while, however, accumulating patches only deadens our sensitivity and our capacity to love freely. Resenting the pain involved in becoming vulnerable to another person causes us to lose heart or harden our heart, and this cuts off the energetic flow between us.

Yet if we can learn to make use of our pain, it can be an invaluable helper and guide on the path. For it exposes and directs our attention to places inside us where we are shut down, contracted, and half-asleep. If I can move with my pain more fluidly, my rigid defenses start to dissolve and I become more permeable to love's awakening influence. And when I can let my partner see my hurt, instead of hiding it away, where it may fester and poison the relationship, this creates greater intimacy between us.

Of course, nobody *wants* to feel pain. Yet to become a warrior of the heart—one who is willing to risk being wounded in the service of love—we must be able to use the pain that relationship inevitably brings our way.

DISILLUSIONMENT AS A STEPPING-STONE

In promoting expectations of unending bliss and security, the dream of love sets us up for shock and disillusionment when we come down to earth and encounter the pain and difficulty involved in creating a satisfying relationship. When these expectations are not fulfilled, it is easy to become bitter and discouraged, with oneself, with the opposite sex, or with love itself.

This was certainly true for Tracy, a woman in her late thirties who had been through many painful disappointments with men. She had grown up assuming that a man would come along one day who would naturally want to take care of her and start a family with her, and that she would, of course, live happily ever after. Yet her life had turned out very differently: No man she had ever wanted had been willing to commit to a relationship with her; she had had to support herself financially; and she was now facing the dreaded biological clock, fearing she might never have a family at all.

Yet at those times when relationships fail to live up to our high-flying dreams and we fall to earth with a jolt, life may actually be giving us a gift—by trying to wake us up. Disillusionment—the recognition that reality does not match our fantasies—is an inevitable and important part of love's path. By bringing us into alignment with the way things are, it can open our eyes to the truth of our situation and help us move in more healthy, positive directions. This can be a real gift, as artist Carla Needleman points out:

> Disillusionment is an extraordinarily interesting state of being, having immediate and far-reaching effects. It is a sacred state that has power. The experience of disillusion stops thought. This has the effect of bringing about in my whole organism a quiet and seriousness that unite me as nothing else has the power to. Only then the mind is receptive and can experience a moment of more precise knowledge.

As long as Tracy tried to ward off her heartache, she was unavailable to the "more precise knowledge" that her disillusion offered. What she needed to do instead was to let herself fall, and then listen to what her pain might have to tell her. Often the endings of significant relationships provide an opportunity for this kind of "descent" into our depths. If we fight our pain and try to "ascend" again too quickly, we will have to face its lessons even more intensely later on. Opening to the grief of disappointment and loss, and letting ourselves go through it, allows old dysfunctional structures to dissolve and new wisdom to enter.

Tracy's disillusionment with relationships offered her a glimpse of certain truths that could help her mobilize herself and move beyond despair: No one else could save her from feeling her aloneness or her wounds from the past. Intimate relationships cannot in themselves heal the basic ache of being a separate individual. No one else could ever provide all the healing love, security, or nurturance she dreamed of. It was futile to seek from a man the confidence she lacked or the love she wouldn't give herself. Painful as these realizations were, they grounded Tracy in reality and gave her a path: She needed to connect with herself more deeply and develop her own strength and confidence, instead of waiting for a man to bring these qualities into her life.

After taking these lessons to heart, Tracy eventually found

what seemed to be a more promising relationship. Yet within a few months, she discovered that her partner was not everything she had hoped he would be. She had discovered some things about him that she strongly disliked, such as a self-centered tightness in his energy. Ordinarily at this point she would have started to close down and protect herself. Yet this time it was different. Even though Mark was not the answer to all her dreams, something inside her would not let her close down so quickly. She felt a fresh, deep quality in their connection that she did not want to throw away. She wanted to try to keep going, to stay open to him just when she felt most tempted to turn away.

BREAKING THE HEART OPEN

Every relationship contains many such moments when we are unable to get what we want or resolve some difference with our partner. Or when we rub up against hurtful, ugly, or contracted places in ourselves or the other that we cannot stand. In truth, we all have certain tendencies that our intimate partners will find it hard to be with, no matter how delightful or highly developed we may be in other areas. Even in the best of relationships, two individuals will never fit together perfectly. There will always be rough edges and problems that cannot be entirely resolved. Because we are creatures of this earth, with all the limitations and imperfections that entails, human relationships cannot always manifest the perfect, unconditional love we know and feel in our heart.

When we feel the pain of this contradiction between the perfect love in our heart and the obstacles to its complete realization in earthly form, it breaks the heart—*wide open*. But this is not so bad. Not so bad at all. When the heart breaks open, we hurt. Yet in this pain is our basic openness to life. When we feel raw and tender, we are in touch with the very core of who we are.

In truth, the heart can never break, for it is already by nature soft and receptive. What actually breaks open is the defensive shell around the heart that we have constructed to try to protect our soft spot, where we feel most deeply affected by life. When this is exposed, we feel the vivid presence of reality as never before.

I am not suggesting that we should just let ourselves suffer instead of trying to improve our relations with our partner. Often our dissatisfactions can play an important role in bringing problem areas to light or in convincing those we love to make changes in their behavior. Yet sooner or later we inevitably discover that the one we love cannot give us everything, be everything we would like, or understand us perfectly. Nor can we ourselves be the ideal prince or princess. What we *can* always do, whenever we encounter the imperfections in our partner or ourselves, is to let them break our heart (open), and let our heart keep expanding, until it can embrace the painful reality we are facing.

When our heart breaks out of the protective shell we have built around it, and we shed our ideal images of how a relationship should be, we may feel naked. Yet in this nakedness we taste the essential nature of our existence. The truth is that we have no ultimate control over what happens to us in this life. Therefore, to feel naked and vulnerable is to be in direct contact with reality. This puts us in touch with ourselves and with our partner in a much deeper way.

BEING WITH PAIN

How then can we open to the pain we feel when reality suddenly dashes our fondest hopes or when our partner does not give us what we want? Often we go numb so that we do not have to feel the pain of our disappointment, or else we passively endure it. Yet nothing much ever comes from trying to ignore our pain, or from suffering stoically. We need to find the inner strength that will allow us to be with our pain in a more active way. We all have this capacity; it is only a question of arousing it. If we can suffer our pain more consciously, it can be of great use to us on our path.

When Carl discovered one day that his partner had slept with another man, his pain was overwhelming. He and Sarah had been together for five years, and this was the longest-lasting relationship he had ever been in. Before Sarah, he had never been willing to commit to a single woman. Whenever he encountered difficulties with previous partners, he had dealt with them by going outside the relationship, seeking out other women. This had allowed him to remain safe and avoid addressing his own problems with intimacy. But now his worst fear had come true: He had been betrayed.

Carl's first impulse was to close his heart to Sarah and turn away from her. However, when he tried to cut off his feelings, he only created a much worse form of suffering—living with a closed heart, feeling half-dead, and lacking motivation to do much of anything. Yet keeping his heart open left him susceptible to an excruciating pain that he did not know how to handle.

In facing intense pain, it is often helpful at first to spend some time making a space for it, allowing it just to be there, "sitting on the edge of it," and inquiring into it (e.g., "What really hurts the most in here?"). Since opening to our pain can be scary, talking about it with someone we love or trust may help us begin to connect with it in this way. As we become more comfortable sitting with our pain, we can let it touch us more directly.

In working with Carl, I tried to help him stay present with how he was feeling in the moment, without either trying to fix the situation or going into despair about it. This put him directly in touch with his pain, and as it flowed through him, he felt as though all his old reference points were being swept away. Often the best way to move through such intense feelings without harming ourselves is to let the heart break open, like a dam bursting, at those moments when we would most like to close it down. When we open to pain that has been dammed up, it feels like riding the rapids of a raging river. *The only way to navigate these rapids is to yield to the energetic flow of the pain.*

Usually we resist doing this because we imagine that it will lead to irreparable harm or destruction. Yet setting ourselves in opposition to pain, as though it were "other," only makes us hard and bitter. If we can open to it, we find not a demon, but *ourselves.* And when we can let it flow freely like the blood in our veins, this clears our system as nothing else can.

Connecting with his pain and following its energetic flow forced Carl to let go of control and his "cool" self-image. This also enabled him to see his situation more clearly. He began to realize that his pain was not just about being betrayed. On a deeper level, it was also a sorrow about never having given himself fully to a relationship. In opening to this sorrow, he saw all the ways that he had kept himself apart from Sarah, just as he had with women all his life. His pain was forcing him to come to terms with his karma—those patterns of fear and denial that had made it impossible for him to have a truly satisfying relationship.

So instead of destroying him, his broken heart was transforming him. Through *opening his heart to his own pain,* he discovered a great warrior spirit that had lain dormant within him most of his life. He became more pliant, and felt more in touch with himself and the beauty of the earth than he had ever been before.

In softening to his pain, Carl also began to empathize more fully with Sarah and appreciate how hard it had been for her to live with him. (Compassion—literally, "suffering-with"—is born out of feeling the rawness of the heart, which also makes us more sensitive to others.) Sarah felt deeply moved when she saw that he was willing to face his pain and be transformed by it. Feeling how much more approachable he was, and sensing a new warmth starting to emanate from him, she found new interest in trying to work on their relationship.

Carl had broken Sarah's heart by not being fully available all those years, and she had broken his by having an affair with another man. All the pain they had been through together—when they eventually shared it with each other in a loving, open way—helped them to connect at a much deeper level than ever before. They realized that their relationship had a larger purpose and significance. Beyond just fulfilling their desires, it was breaking them open. A couple will find that they can go through many heartbreaks together—without losing heart—if they can use them in this way, as path.

VULNERABILITY AND GENTLENESS

When we first open to our pain, it often feels as though we are bleeding. Yet this kind of emotional bleeding helps awaken the heart, allowing vital energies in us that have become coagulated to circulate again. To let our pain move in this healing way requires awareness, courage, and gentleness—being present with the pain instead of believing scare stories in our mind about where it might take us, opening ourselves to the place where we hurt inside, bringing a caring presence to it, and letting those we love see it as well. In this way, by helping us connect with our warrior spirit, pain can become a friend and ally.

Thus when Tracy fully felt her disappointment that Mark wasn't everything she would like him to be, and let this touch her, she realized, "We each have differences and imperfections that hurt each other. Yet there is nothing wrong with feeling that pain. It makes me feel my heart's blood—my openness to myself, to him, and to love itself." In proclaiming her vulnerability in this way, Tracy was stepping beyond her fear of pain and heartbreak.

Unfortunately, the word *vulnerability* has a pejorative meaning in our culture. Associating it with weakness and powerlessness, we often think of a vulnerable person as someone who is overly sensitive to being hurt or offended. Yet sensitivity to offense is something quite different from the genuine vulnerability of letting our heart be exposed. The ego is always fragile and easily wounded. It is a brittle shell or facade, a pretense that we are "in charge," that no one can "get to us," that we are "captains of our fate." It is fragile because life is always threatening to expose our pretense of having power *over* life. By contrast, acknowledging our basic human vulnerability—our openness to reality—is a source of real power. In fearlessly allowing ourselves to be vulnerable, we embody the bravery and gentleness of a true warrior.

Always before, Tracy had tried to make her partners meet her emotional needs in devious, indirect ways. She would avoid stating her real feelings and needs openly because she did not like to feel exposed. It was much safer to manipulate her partner into giving, blame him when he failed to do so, or just withdraw.

In every relationship, there are times when one partner wants to connect more deeply, but the other is not as emotionally available at the same moment. At first when Tracy experienced this with Mark, she would feel hurt, and then contract, protect herself, attack, or hold it against him. Then, as her hurt and resentment built up, she would start to think about leaving him. Yet in learning to be compassionate toward the vulnerable part of herself where she felt hurt by Mark's unavailability, Tracy could let these hard, defensive edges fall away. When she softened to her pain, she could simply tell Mark about it, instead of holding it against him or shutting down her love. Expressing her needs more openly, rather than manipulating or accusing him, allowed her love to keep flowing. And she felt stronger: no longer did she have to live in fear of pain or feel victimized when she got hurt. In this way, through making friends with our vulnerability, we discover a new kind of flexibility and power.

We usually think of vulnerability and gentleness as the opposite of power. Yet the softening that happens when we work with our pain can be quite compelling and influential. We become like water, which can generate electric power precisely because it flows so willingly, without resisting gravity or the contours of the land. Water is extremely vulnerable, in a sense. It is soft, it does not resist the touch, it can be molded into any shape, and it receives whatever we put into it. Yet for wearing down what is hard and tough, nothing surpasses it. Just as water, which is so soft and accommodating, can reduce the hardest of rocks to sand, similarly gentleness is one of the most irresistible human qualities and can penetrate even the hardest of hearts.

Whereas hardness stirs up aggression, gentleness provides nothing to resist.

So when Tracy could show her vulnerability by saying, "I want to feel close to you right now," or "I just need to feel your love," Mark could not resist her. Because she was so appealing at that moment, he would often *want* to put aside his self-involvement and give her what she asked for. And when she could expose her pain—"It really hurts me when you get so tight"—instead of trying to get him to change, this usually made him soften. No longer was she the fussy princess expecting him to be the perfect prince.

In learning to appreciate and trust her broken-open heart, Tracy felt more connected with life than ever before, and more capable of handling the challenges of an ongoing relationship. This was a tremendous victory, which only made her stronger and more attractive.

Men particularly have a hard time seeing that their willingness to be vulnerable is often what touches women the most. They imagine that it is a sign of weakness, and that it will lead to scorn or rejection. However, as one woman friend of mine put it, "I find it quite magnetic when a man lets me see his vulnerability. It only turns me off if he tries to get me to reassure him about feeling that way. If he just presents it openly, I find that courageous and admire him for it." What she is saying is that ego fragility—trying to cover up the rawness of one's heart—is unattractive, while fearlessly revealing it can be most appealing.

THE MYSTERY OF LOVE

Thus the rawness of the broken-open heart, which begins in moments of disillusion, is the transmuting force in the alchemy of love. When we let our heart break open, a certain sweetness starts to flow from us like nectar. As the Sufi teacher Hazrat Inayat Khan put it, "The warmth of the lover's atmosphere, the piercing effect of his voice, the appeal of his words, all come from the pain of his heart." This is one of the great secrets of love. Instead of trying to ward off this pain, which is futile anyway, the lover can use it to transform himself, to develop invincible tenderness and compassion, and, as the troubadours discovered, become a "gentle man" as well as a heroic warrior in the service of love.

Letting the heart break open awakens us to the mystery of love—that we can't help loving others, in spite of the pain they cause us, for no other reason than that they move and touch us, in ways that we can never fully comprehend. Indeed, if those we love perfectly matched our ideal dreams, they would not touch us so deeply. What we love is not just their pure being, but also their heart's struggle with all the obstacles in the way of its full, radiant expression. Although their imperfections cause us pain, they also give our love a greater purchase, a foothold, something to work with. It is as though our heart wants to ally itself with the heart in those we love and lend them strength in their struggle to realize the magnificence of their being, beyond all their perceived shortcomings. So, just as rocks in a stream accentuate the force of the water rushing against them, the obstacles to perfect romance can help us realize the power of our capacity to love. They force the heart to stretch so that it can embrace all of what we are. This, more than finding the perfect relationship or having someone give us everything we want, is what can heal us.

8

Conscious Commitment

WHEN WE FIRST FALL IN LOVE, our experience is so compelling that we can easily overlook potential problems in a relationship. Yet when these later prove difficult or hard to handle, we need something more than just inspiration. This is where the question of commitment comes in. Commitment means choosing to work with those obstacles that interfere with the free flow of love, both in ourselves and in the relationship.

Yet it is no longer as clear as it once was just why two people should vow to stay together and persevere when problems and obstacles arise between them. We have few examples of what a healthy, alive commitment between two people would look like. The old model—based on *duty*—makes commitment into a kind of glue. So many of our parents "stuck it out for the kids" or for fear of family disapproval at the expense of their growth, integrity, and freedom that it is hardly surprising if the notion of long-term commitment rouses no great enthusiasm among the younger generations today. At the other extreme, many couples decide to marry out of idealistic *hope,* without carefully considering what they are getting in for. They imagine that their romantic feelings will be enough to keep them going. Then, when their grace period runs out and conflicts arise, they are unprepared to deal with the situation.

In former times, commitment was defined and imposed on a couple by society and family. In a traditional arranged marriage, a man and a woman would have to vow to stay together forever before even getting to know each other. With this kind of background, it is not surprising that so much unconsciousness surrounds commitment today, and that many of us stumble into marriage half-asleep. Now that external pressures no longer enforce or sustain a couple's commitment, a more conscious approach is called for.

Staying together is but a small part of what genuine commitment entails, only the outer expression of an inner dedication. The essence of a living commitment is *two people's devotion to their mutual unfolding,* which can only be based on a more primary commitment within each individual to open more fully to life itself.

Initially, two partners cannot be sure what they are doing together or how far their relationship can go. Yet through testing the power of their connection—the depth of their love and their capacity to handle its challenges—they become clearer about its place in their lives, and can thus honor and affirm it more wholeheartedly. Instead of starting out as a promise—"till death do us part"—spoken at the marriage altar, conscious commitment is something that develops more gradually. It is a more advanced stage of a relationship that evolves out of successfully navigating many earlier tests and challenges. Such a commitment is awake and alive. Unlike something manufactured out of duty, hope, or preconceived ideas, it emerges organically from the relationship's own ripening, and is full of passion, freshness, and spontaneity—the very juice of love.

STEPS TOWARD A CONSCIOUS COMMITMENT*

1. Making a Genuine Connection

The ground of a strong and lasting commitment is the passionate connection between two people whose beings say yes to each other. When two people connect being-to-being, they experience a deep "soul-resonance" that goes beyond mere romance or desire. Something powerful and real inside them starts waking up and coming alive in each other's presence. It is often surprising because they cannot reason themselves into or out of it. Although it seems to arise mysteriously out of nowhere, it may also have a certain familiarity, as one woman described in her connection with her husband:

> I felt when I met him that I had known him before, as if for many lifetimes. I especially remember waking up next to him with the profound feeling that I had just woken up after a thousand years.

Just as the body of a guitar amplifies and enriches the vibration of the strings to produce a full, rich musical sound, similarly, the resonance between two beings amplifies and enriches the qualities of each. This kind of "soul-connection" can sustain two people much longer than attraction to each other's personalities or attributes. Out of this passionate resonance grows a devotion to each other's unfolding—which can allow them to persevere through difficult times and overcome any obstacles that threaten to come between them.

2. Testing the Connection: Working with Whatever Arises

The deeper a soul-connection goes, however, the more it brings our karmic patterns and personal neuroses to the surface. So

*I present these important steps along the way, not as an ideal or exact prescription, but as a framework to encourage you to explore this path more fully for yourself.

before two people can feel confident about making a commitment to each other, they need to find out whether they can handle this challenge.

The penetrating quality of an honest, loving connection wears away our facades, bringing out the best and the worst in us. Along with our openheartedness, all our fears, insecurities, and resistances to intimacy start to emerge. We may find ourselves becoming more emotional, jealous, or unreasonable than we had ever thought possible. We may discover new intensities of terror. We may recoil in horror at all the hard, tight, petty places we come up against inside ourselves. And we may seriously doubt whether we have what it takes to make a go of relationship at all. Real intimacy, in short, brings up our unfinished business—all the rough spots in ourselves and in our partner that still need to be polished, refined, and further developed.

So, although many couples marry purely out of delight in each other, it may be better for two people to go through a certain amount of disappointment, heartbreak, and strife before making such a commitment. Such experiences provide a way of testing themselves and their relationship. Can they handle the disappointment of realizing that they can never meet all of each other's needs? Does their relationship depend on a limited set of roles—he as commanding, she as yielding, for example—or can they make room for all their different sides? Can they include not just their sweetness and love, but also the thunderstorms that arise between them?

The main question facing a couple when they come up against their rough edges is, can they work with whatever arises between them, no matter how demanding it may be, and include that as part of their path together? *Working with* whatever arises means *facing it and meeting it with their attention and concern, so that they can find a way to move through it.* If they cannot do this, they can never be fully present in the relationship, and therefore never fully committed.

Couples often have to face this test early on in their relationship. For example, after Nicole spent a wonderful first two months of getting to know Phillip, she discovered that he had an overbearing "steamroller" side that often left her feeling trampled into the ground. He in turn felt disappointed that she did not stand her ground and engage with him more forcefully. At first they avoided dealing with these discontents because they were uncertain whether any good would come of it. Nicole did not know whether Phillip could hear or respond to her need for more gentleness and consideration, while he wondered whether she had any interest in becoming more powerful. Until they could answer these questions, they could not move any closer. Fortunately for their relationship, they were each willing to work with the obstacles that were preventing a fuller connection between them. This provided an important early test of how far they could go together.

We do not necessarily fail at "working with" just because we want to run away from difficulties. We *will* want to run away sometimes. That is to be expected. In working with their differences, two partners can expect to experience moments of intense frustration with each other when they will be tempted to give up. The important question is not whether we go away sometimes, *but whether we come back.* Although we may never be able to handle everything that comes along perfectly, it is the *intention* to face what is happening that allows a relationship to keep moving forward.

3. Forging a Container: Including All of Who We Are

In working with what comes up between them, two partners begin to find out just how large their relationship can be. If it is a narrow box they have to squeeze into, it will not promote their unfolding. Their commitment can nurture their growth only if it is a spacious container that can accommodate all the different ways they are. So, as they begin to work with difficulties, further testing occurs, to determine whether they can include the whole of themselves in their relationship.

Forging a strong, healthy relationship container involves learning to *accommodate*—or make a friendly space for—whatever feelings arise between ourselves and our partner. This does not mean that we should always like our feelings, much less act them out. Instead, it means giving ourselves and each other permission *to feel what we feel,* instead of ignoring or criticizing it.

The process of accommodating feelings in a relationship involves working out a balance between *containment and expression.* Consciously containing feelings means bringing attention to them, giving them space, and seeing what they have to tell us. Impulsively expressing everything we feel or venting emotions because we are uncomfortable containing them will eventually overwhelm our partner, thereby constricting and shutting down communication. If that is our usual style, then our work involves learning to contain our feelings and work with them inside ourselves. This is important because there is always more to a feeling than what is at first apparent. Anger is never *just* anger. Underneath it, we may discover hurt or disappointment, or perhaps a clear message that is important to deliver to our partner. Containing the anger helps us to see what more is in it. When we work with our feelings first, our words have more power when we do express them. They become a form of communication rather than an assault.

Yet if our typical style is not to express feelings, this also limits and constricts how fully we can connect with our partner. If we withdraw into ourselves every time something hurts us or makes us angry, whole areas of interaction become closed off. Our work then involves learning to open up and become more expressive.

A major obstacle to accommodating difficult feelings is the belief that we shouldn't have them in the first place. For example, one young man I worked with felt overwhelmed by the strain of the arrival of his firstborn child, but he fought against acknowledging his fears, because they contradicted his image of "How A Real Man Should Be." He also wondered whether his wife would still love him if he revealed these feelings. To work with the situation, Peter had to first make space for his feeling of "I can't handle this," instead of blaming himself for it. When he could do this, it took the pressure off and allowed him to consider more calmly what was going on. In giving himself room to feel upset, he discovered important information that he needed to recognize and communicate: He was feeling neglected by his wife, and needed to take better care of himself as well.

Doing this inner work—connecting with his feelings, caring for them, and giving them space—was the essential groundwork that then allowed Peter to talk constructively with Diane about the situation. If he had just blurted out his raw feelings ("I'm upset and want to get away; I hate it that you're spending so much time with the baby") he would have only made her defensive. Instead, by containing his feelings first, he got to know them better. This allowed him to express himself more clearly and skillfully: "I've been having a hard time, wondering whether I can handle all this, and that scares me. I want to be a good husband and father, but I'm really feeling stressed out. And I'm concerned about how little quality time we have together anymore."

This communication evoked Diane's empathy. However, since it also aroused her fears, she too needed room to acknowledge her feelings. By creating a space together in which they could share the pain and difficulty of their situation, along with their deepest fears, they grew closer than they had been since the baby was born. Thus the very feelings that at first seem most threatening can actually promote deeper intimacy, if two partners can accommodate and share them openly.

Unfortunately, what happens more typically in relationships is that one partner shuts down when the other tries to express difficult feelings. Grant had fallen in love with Teresa because of some very warm and open moments they had shared. Yet as they grew closer, Teresa's old fears about intimacy began to surface. When she tried to tell Grant about them, he felt angry and disappointed. Instead of letting her know how he felt, he nursed his anger in private and distanced himself from her. As a result, they began to grow apart.

Even between the closest of couples, feelings will arise that

make them feel separate or distant. What we often do not realize, however, is that communicating about obstacles to intimacy
can itself be a vital form of intimacy. Ironically, Grant's preconceived notion of "how intimacy should be" kept him from allowing his partner to have her real feelings; his belief that if she
loved him she should be more open precluded greater openness
between them. He did not see the potential path here—that
making room for their different feelings could create greater
closeness between them.

When they came in for counseling, I tried to help Grant see
that if he wanted greater intimacy, he would have to make room
not only for Teresa's fear, but also for his own responses to it.
This was a revelation for him. He had not realized that he could
tell her, "When you get scared and pull back, I feel tremendously sad and disappointed. I'm afraid I'm losing a love that
feels really healing to me." Yet when he finally could say this,
it evoked Teresa's empathy and gave her more room to share
her fears as well—and this allowed her to move closer again.
When two partners can accommodate their feelings in this way,
they gain confidence that they can include the whole of themselves in their relationship. This naturally increases their sense
of commitment.

For two people to include all of themselves in a relationship
means walking a thin line, neither suppressing how they are nor
just indulging their habitual patterns. In considering how to
work with Phillip's steamroller tendencies, Nicole realized that
she could not just reject this part of him because it also contained a fiery intensity essential to who he was. Other than the
aggressive way it sometimes came across, she actually found his
fieriness attractive. Realizing this helped her find the right balance—letting him know that she liked his intensity, but that it
hurt her when he overpowered her with it. Since she was not
trying to suppress his basic fieriness, and was willing to expose
the pain it sometimes caused her, Phillip could hear what she
had to say. Seeing how important this was for her and for the
good of their relationship, he could respond positively, without
becoming defensive or aggressive.

If Nicole had attacked or condemned Phillip for the way he was, he might have promised to change, out of guilt. Yet trying to cut off part of ourselves for the sake of our partner never works. A basic law of the psyche is that whatever we try to exclude from consciousness will keep trying to regain entry, until we recognize and include it as part of who we are. If we reject some part of ourselves, regarding it as alien and unacceptable, then when it does find a way in, it will often rebound on us in a way that wreaks havoc. When Phillip's aggression did surface again, it probably would have taken an even harsher form.

All too often we imagine that we must bend ourselves out of shape to fit into a relationship. For instance, we might think, "Now that I am married, I shouldn't feel any longing for independence, for being alone, or for other deep, intimate friendships." Yet no matter how committed we are to a relationship, we will continue to feel desires to be alone and attractions to other people. If we try to eliminate such feelings, they will only haunt us, making us regard the relationship as a prison. Or they may suddenly erupt as an irresistible urge to run off and have an affair. If commitment becomes a glue that keeps us stuck in feeling only one way, eventually we will feel the urge to break free of it.

We need a more expansive view of commitment—as a journey of two people learning to open more fully to life, through working with the whole of who they are. Then, whatever feelings arise can be seen as an integral part of their journey, and need not threaten their relationship. Just as we might pacify a wild horse by giving it a large pasture in which to roam about, so we can make room for all our different feelings in a relationship. When we don't fight them, they gradually relax, and then we can learn to ride them instead of being carried away by them. Often we imagine that commitment means suppressing our wild feelings through coercive or restrictive measures. Yet if we try to stamp out the wildness in ourselves or in others, we only give it something to fight against. We may also wind up killing off our passion, which is an expression of this wild energy.

One happily married man I know was unclear about how to handle the passion he sometimes felt for other women. Suppressing these feelings only undermined his male vitality, which also had negative consequences for his connection with his wife. Yet could he let himself feel them? Could she handle it if he did? As a couple, he and his wife had to work on expanding the container of their relationship to include their feelings for other people. They finally agreed that they needed to make room for these feelings, and that this was not the same as acting them out. This allowed their passion to keep circulating freely, contributing to the life and health of their relationship.

It can be especially hard to accommodate our need to say no in a relationship. If we imagine that commitment means *only* saying yes, we may feel guilty about saying no to someone we love. Instead of saying no directly, we may say it indirectly or deviously, by going along with something halfheartedly or withholding ourselves in some way. Yet every place we are afraid of acknowledging our no is a place where we withdraw energy from the relationship and avoid genuine contact.

No has an essential place in any relationship. As an expression of our individuality and difference from our partner, it helps keep the spark of passion alive. We cannot say yes wholeheartedly unless we can also say no. When we are free to say either yes or no, then we can bring the whole of ourselves into the relationship, and this promotes stronger commitment.

Often we say yes just to avoid a fight. Yet there can be real energy and power in saying no to someone face-to-face, without apology or pretense, and without breaking contact. When my partner stands up to me or asserts her truth in this way, it deepens my respect for her.

If saying no leads to a fight, that is not necessarily bad. The fiery, angry energy arising out of the friction between two strong individuals can often help them break through barriers and work out important issues between them. Anger is problematic only when we use it as a weapon of blame or attack.

One of the great challenges in every relationship is learning to express anger cleanly, as simple, direct communication.

Doing this can often help a couple reestablish contact when they have grown distant. One creative way to express anger, without doing harm, is through "whimsical rascality." Playfully wrestling or teasing, for example, can transform aggression into humor. When we can be playful with our anger, it conveys a spark of vitality, rather than just combativeness. Burning cleanly, it leaves no residue of resentment or smoldering rage.

A DANGER: CRITIC STORIES

What often makes it hard to accommodate feelings is that we interpret them as a sign of something wrong with us. In so doing, we turn against ourselves and give in to our "critic"— that scolding, attacking inner voice that continually focuses on what is wrong and tells us we are never good enough. Couples often panic at their own or each other's feelings, and construct ominous stories that act as self-fulfilling prophecies. So it is essential for every couple to learn to distinguish stories—their mental fabrications, judgments, or interpretations, which they then treat as reality—from their feelings. Then when difficult emotions arise, they can work with them directly, instead of becoming carried away or intimidated by gloom-and-doom stories.

Peter's initial belief—that because he felt so much conflict about his new baby, he must be a horrible person—is an example of a story told by the critic. In truth, Peter's feeling of being overwhelmed did not mean that there was something wrong with him; it was simply a signal to pay attention to some pressing needs. Diane also could have made up a critic story, out of her anxiety, concluding that Peter was unreliable and that their marriage was in danger. This would have prevented her from hearing what was really going on for him. If she had blamed him for his feelings, she would have further activated his own critic, which would have caused him to contract and feel all the more overwhelmed. And this could have set in motion a sequence of events that might well have led to the disastrous conclusion she imagined.

Unless a couple recognize this kind of dynamic, they may

wind up unconsciously forging a "critic alliance." For instance, a man's critic may be in league with the woman's critic to keep her down. Whenever she "gets out of line," his critic chimes in, which causes her critic to give her a verbal beating and bring her back into line.

A relationship can serve our growth so powerfully because it reveals our stuck patterns more vividly than most other situations in our lives. As these patterns come to light, it is easy to start attacking ourselves, or blaming our partner for the powerful emotions that may be released. Yet imagining that our feelings mean something about what kind of person we are only solidifies them further. Feeling anger does not mean that I am an aggressive person. Feeling vulnerable does not mean that I am weak. Feeling fear about giving does not mean that I am hopelessly selfish. If we can see the volatility of our feelings as a sign that a relationship is deeply affecting us and shaking loose old karmic patterns, we can let them arise and pass through us without condemning ourselves for them.

So if I feel anger or fear with my partner, I can always use such feelings as path by inquiring into them: "I'm angry and scared—what does this mean? What is happening underneath these feelings? What is so scary?" Perhaps I find that I am jealous of my partner's strength in an area where I am weak. I see that I am afraid of being judged as a complete bungler in an area where she excels. But if I put aside my self-critical stories, then I can see that I have something to learn from her, and this helps me open myself to the situation again.

As two lovers work with what comes up between them, make room for all the different sides of themselves, and accommodate their difficult feelings, a real trust can start to grow up between them. Then they can say, with honesty and humor, "I have seen all your tricks, and I want to go forward with you, including all that." This kind of trust is different from the naive faith of "Because we love each other, I know you'll never hurt me." Such blind faith is foolish, because there are parts of everyone that are *not* trustworthy. Genuine trust develops between two people, not because everything about them is trustworthy, but because they can work with all the different parts of themselves, including those that are not trustworthy.

As a couple's commitment grows, it becomes like an alchemical vessel, in which all the karmic patterns that cloud their full radiant expression can be held and healed within love's larger embrace. The heat of their connection can transform these patterns into the gold of authentic being. Although they may have seen flashes of this gold in the first rush of love, working with all the different sides of each other allows it to shine through more brightly.

4. Going Beyond "Me First"

Intimate relationships always ask us to give up something we cherish: certain favorite privacies, preferences, or ways of staying securely defended. They require us to take a leap beyond our usual style of defending our personal territory. So a further step in the development of an organic commitment is for a couple to explore their willingness to come out of hiding and leave behind old egocentric attitudes and behavior.

Going beyond a "me first" attitude involves relaxing the demands and expectations I place on my partner, expanding my concern for her well-being, and becoming more sensitive to the needs of the relationship as a whole, beyond what just feels personally safe and comfortable. In giving up territory and caring for my partner's well-being, I start to cast in my lot with her. I am no longer the sole center of my life.

Those of us who find going beyond a "me first" attitude difficult may be tempted to choose a way of life other than a committed relationship. Yet if we deeply examine what is most important and satisfying in life, we may find that we feel most alive when we can step out of the confines of our usual self-absorption. The Russian theologian Solovyov wrote that erotic love is the most powerful means for overcoming our usual habit of ascribing absolute significance exclusively to ourselves, while denying it to others. Recognizing the absolute significance of this *other* we love, who is wholly different from us, expands our horizons and opens us more fully to life as a whole.

5. Developing a Vision and Making a Choice

The more two people help each other work with whatever arises, include the whole of themselves in their relationship, and expand their boundaries, the more they appreciate how they are serving each other's unfolding. This helps them develop a clear vision of what they are doing together—which in turn allows them to make a conscious choice to be together.

It is odd how many people wind up married without ever having consciously chosen to be in a committed relationship, and remain in the marriage halfheartedly, forever finding reasons for complaint and dissatisfaction. So it is important to see clearly what commitment involves and, if that is what we want, to choose it as a way of life. Then whatever difficulties arise can become part of our journey rather than reasons to complain or bail out.

In former times, society and family conceived and held the vision of the man/woman relationship. Yet now that our society provides dream-fantasies instead of workable guidelines, each couple must forge their own vision to guide and inspire them to keep moving forward. A vision that develops out of testing their relationship and seeing how they further each other's unfolding is a much stronger bond than any hope or obligation. Vision and conscious choice give us strength to keep going, even in times when our courage or confidence may wane.

COMMITMENT AS PATH

If a couple can remain awake while moving through these stages—making a connection, working with what comes up, including all the different sides of themselves, going beyond "me first," and forging a vision—their commitment will naturally be more conscious. If you trace what went wrong in a previous relationship or marriage that did not work out for you, you will probably find that you got involved in it *without really knowing what you were doing.* Either your connection was not that strong to begin with, or else you did not know how to work with the difficulties that arose. Now imagine doing it differently the next time. You feel a deep, passionate resonance with your partner and you both care about each other's unfolding. You test things out for a couple of years until you are satisfied that you can work with whatever comes up and include all of yourself in the relationship. You are both learning to give of yourselves and stretch your boundaries. You develop a strong vision about why you are together. In such a case, what would prevent you from sharing a life together?

Conscious commitment is a pact between beings, rather than between personalities. In effect, my partner and I say to each other, "Whatever problems our personalities have together, we will not let them get between us. If our egos are at war, we will not let that ruin our deeper connection—we will always come back and meet on this deeper level. We will help each other wake up and become all that we can be. We will keep opening to each other and to life itself in and through this relationship." Without such an alliance between our beings, our egos will likely conspire to perpetuate old habitual patterns, and the container we create may become a prison or a hollow shell. Conscious commitment is to *being* together, not just staying together.

Of course, two partners may connect deeply on the being level, yet still be unable to work things out on the personality level. That is why the testing stage is so important. If they cannot find ways to work on things together, it means that their personality conflicts are more powerful than their being-connection. Therefore they cannot move toward greater commitment.

When Orage, a student of the Russian teacher Gurdjieff, wrote that a great love can both take hold and let go, he was expressing the earth and heaven of conscious commitment. Letting go means creating a large open space in which we can let ourselves and our partner be, as we are. Taking hold means working with whatever comes up in that space. Yet if working on the relationship becomes too serious and earthbound, it will weigh a couple down. Just as a plant that is overfertilized will wilt, so a relationship that is fussed over too much will suffer. This is where letting go can provide balance, often through humor. We can create plenty of room in a relationship to kid ourselves and each other, and laugh at the gap between our lofty ideals and how we actually are. Conscious commitment keeps us awake, for it involves continually finding our balance on the edge of taking hold and letting go.

Above all, it is important not to be too idealistic about all this, force anything on ourselves, or try to be ahead of where we really are. Approaching commitment as a "should" only makes us go unconscious, setting us up for further difficulties or failures. There is a Tibetan saying: "Knowledge must be burned, hammered, and beaten like pure gold. Then one can wear it as an ornament." In the same vein, we could say: "Commitment must be burned, hammered, and beaten like pure gold. Then it can display itself as marriage."

Those of us who undertake this journey are having to learn something new—how to let commitment evolve naturally, through many ups and downs, steps forward and back. So our uncertainty about whether we can handle all the challenges along the way is not a problem. *For it is part of the path itself.* I was heartened in this regard by the words of Chögyam Trungpa, a Tibetan teacher who was once asked how he managed to escape the Chinese invasion, trekking across the snowbound Himalayas, with little preparation, supplies, or assurance about the route or the outcome. His reply was brief: "One foot after the other."

9

Obstacles on the Path

OPENING OUR HEART TO ANOTHER, as we have seen, eventually brings us up against the obstacles to love inside us—all the contracted places where we fear intimacy or want to stay closed. Soon we find ourselves acting out the same old self-defeating games we have been caught in all our lives, and this leads to struggle and conflict with our partner. Commitment involves a decision to work with these fears and rigid patterns that arise in a relationship. Yet to work effectively with them, we also need to recognize what we are up against. Understanding the forces at work in our struggles with our partner can help us come to grips with them instead of just being at their mercy. Then these obstacles can become stepping-stones that lead forward, rather than barriers that block our way.

FAMILY BACKGROUND AND CONDITIONED PATTERNS

How each of us expresses and receives love in relationships— and fears doing so—was established long ago, in our very first intimate relationships—with our mothers and fathers. Our parents have a tremendous influence over us, not just because our well-being depended so totally on them, but because they were the first people we loved deeply. Unfortunately, our first loves usually leave us with wounds that we carry with us for the rest of our lives.

The psychological influence of parents on children is particularly strong in a society like ours where extended families, tight-knit communities, and initiation rituals, which once mitigated the parents' impact, have broken down or disappeared. Growing up in an isolated nuclear family, apart from a larger kinship network, does not provide enough space from parents or a wide enough range of models of healthy male and female behavior.[1] The parent–child relationship often proves to be either too close or too distant, both of which lead to difficulties in later relationships.

ABANDONMENT AND ENGULFMENT

At the core of all fears of intimacy is a fear of loss. People whose parents were distant or unavailable usually fear loss of love and contact. They are afraid of being neglected or abandoned again. They may cling to relationships in an addictive way, demanding that their partners continually prove their love. Or they may keep one foot out the door so that they are never in a situation where they could be abandoned again.

At the other extreme, children whose parents were too close, invasive, or controlling fear losing *themselves*—their psychological space, which allows them to feel their integrity as individuals. One extreme but common form of parental encroachment on a child's space is "psychic incest," where a mother who is dissatisfied with her husband turns to her son for emotional fulfillment, or a father unconsciously tries to keep his daughter's affections all to himself. These secret pacts between parent and child result in sons feeling emotionally tied to their mothers ("mama's boys") and daughters feeling bound to their fathers ("daddy's little girls"). Those who suffered from invasive parents will fear engulfment—being emotionally controlled or smothered by an intimate partner.

Because relations with parents often contain complex, con-

tradictory influences, many of us grow up fearing both abandonment and engulfment—which get played out differently in different relationships. With one partner we might fight to maintain our separate space, yet with a different partner we may wind
up fighting for greater intimacy and closeness.[2]

When we play out these fears in a relationship, we are
reenacting old scenes from the universal drama of childhood,
which has two main subplots: first bonding with our parents,
then separating from them and becoming an individual in our
own right. Those of us who could not bond deeply with the
parents we loved or separate fully from them leave childhood
wounded in these areas.

Our anxiety about our frustrated needs causes us either
to turn against these parts of ourselves or to exaggerate them.
If our parents did not respond to our need for love and caring,
we will often feel guilty (and/or demanding) about wanting
emotional support and connectedness. Or if our parents did
not value our need to be independent, we may feel guilty
(and/or defiant) about wanting to be a separate individual.
And we perpetuate these kinds of woundedness by maintaining an attitude of conditional self-love that obstructs the free
flow of love in later relationships ("I only like myself *if* I don't
need anyone . . . or *if* I am pleasing to others").

People with abandonment fears often feel ashamed and
disempowered when they desire to connect with others. Since
they do not believe that they can express their need for contact
in a way that will inspire a positive response, they act it out in
devious, distorted, or compulsive ways. They may become demanding, manipulative, or critical when their partner is not
there in the way they want. This usually has the effect of pushing
the partner away—which further frustrates their need for contact and makes them feel even more helpless about ever having
it met.

Furthermore, since they feel chronically starved for affection, it is hard for them to recognize the complementary set of
needs—to spend time alone, to have their own space, and to be
self-contained. Consequently, their partner starts acting out

these needs instead and they polarize into antagonistic, warring positions.

The same situation holds true in reverse for those who fear losing their individuality in a relationship. Because of their childhood experience with invasive or engulfing parents, they feel conflicted about being separate individuals and lack confidence in their autonomy. Thus they act out their need for space and freedom in exaggerated ways, by defensively keeping their distance or pushing their partner away. Since too much intimacy could threaten their already fragile sense of independence, they also cannot fully acknowledge their complementary need for closeness and connectedness. When their partner expresses this need instead, the two of them become locked into a polarized struggle.

In sum, relationships inevitably reactivate old wounds from childhood in the areas of bonding and separating. Our old fears of not getting what we need make us feel powerless when these needs arise in a relationship. This makes us act them out in unfriendly, exaggerated, or manipulative ways, thereby pushing our partner in the other direction. Our partner in turn starts acting out the opposite set of needs, those that we have a hard time acknowledging ourselves. And this leads to an ongoing struggle, whose real nature is often unclear to either of us.

If we continue to act out our wounds unconsciously, they will forever create conflict in our relationships. For they interfere with the flow of the dance of intimacy, which involves moving freely back and forth between "me" and "we"—keeping our seat as a strong, self-contained individual and bonding as a couple.

Fortunately, we *can* begin to heal these wounds—even in the midst of relationships where they are stirring up the most trouble. In fact, one of the great gifts of a deep relationship is that it brings these core wounds to light, thus allowing us to bring attention to them and free ourselves from their influence.

Old wounds continue to control our behavior only because we have withdrawn our awareness from them. Since we have essentially gone to sleep in these places, we must first wake up to how our wounds affect us if we want to free ourselves from their grip. We can do this by using the *external conflicts* they create to develop greater awareness of the *internal conflicts* we feel around our needs. In this way, we can use any struggle with our partner as a path—to help us rediscover and empower the wounded, helpless parts of ourselves where we are blocking the flow of love that could most nourish our development.

STORIES AND SCRIPTS

Yet usually what we do instead is to play out the same self-defeating patterns over and over again. What makes it so hard to see and change what we are doing?

I once worked with a man who would become so obsessed and grasping every time he became involved with a woman that he would soon drive her away. This would leave him feeling hurt, abandoned, and unloved. As a result, he concluded that he was unfit to be in a relationship at all. Why did Chris keep repeating such a destructive pattern, especially when he knew that it got him nowhere?

Underlying all such compulsive behavior is something more persistent: a story or script that we are playing out. Stories are ways in which we try to interpret our experience by ascribing fixed meaning to particular events in our lives. After we tell ourselves a story enough times, it generalizes into a master script that governs the play of our lives. Stories rationalize and perpetuate the wounded, contracted places within us. Instead of saying, "I'm lonely and hurting inside," Scrooge says, "Bah, humbug." If he could simply acknowledge his hurt, he could begin to soften inside and address his unfulfilled needs. But the cover story he invents to hide his wound—"People are fools. Who needs them?"—only solidifies his wound and maintains its hold on him.

In looking into his tendency to grab on to every new relationship, Chris discovered the story he was telling himself: "I'm not really worthy of a wonderful relationship; I can't *have* such wonderful feelings." Since he believed this, the next step was: "Therefore, I'd better grab what I can right now, before this woman disappears." Because he was in such a rush to seize what he believed could never last, he would ignore any proper sense of timing. He would give himself to the relationship immediately, instead of letting it develop naturally. This would scare his partner away, thus confirming his story: "I can't really have this."

Chris's story was part of a master script that he enacted in many different areas of his life: "There is something wrong with me, I'm not enough." Chris had developed this belief as a way of coping with severe deprivation and neglect in childhood. Children typically try to understand why their parents are not more loving by imagining that they themselves are bad and undeserving of love. Thus Chris had come to believe that his parents neglected him because he was not good enough. In so doing, he had solidified his deprivation into an identity. Thus he found a way to make "something"—an identity for himself—out of "nothing"—his unfulfilled needs. This provided a security of sorts, the only kind that was available at the time.

Ever since, Chris felt most fully "himself" when he felt empty, hungry, deprived. As a child, this had been a brilliant strategy for keeping himself together in a family situation that threatened his physical and emotional survival. Yet as an adult, his attachment to this skewed identity made it impossible to receive nourishment from other people. If a woman wanted to give to him, he would feel as though he were losing himself. He could feel like himself only when chasing after her, feeling hungry, or losing her, feeling bereft.

Here are other common examples of stories learned in childhood that set up negative life scripts:

- "I don't deserve love."
- "I have to earn love."
- "I can never get what I really want."
- "I will only be loved if I play hard to get."
- "If others see my need, they'll run away."

- "I don't trust love—it's a form of control."
- "I must save women."
- "I must always be pleasing to men."
- "No one will love me if I show myself as I really am."

Even though these beliefs about love may be unreasonable and harmful, they can be quite persistent. One reason for this is that, despite the pain they cause, they give us a secure sense of identity. This gives them a staying power that defies logic and common sense. One of the most obviously lovable women I have known had a story that she was unlovable, which persisted despite people's nearly universal positive response to her. Born out of the neglect she suffered as a child, this story helped her maintain a defiant stance, which allowed her to feel safe whenever her need for love arose.

Furthermore, we come to believe that our story accurately represents the way things really are. Yet in truth it is only a dream, a conditioned pattern of beliefs that keeps recreating the kind of situation that wounded us in the first place. By determining how we set up our relationships, such stories become self-fulfilling prophecies, recreating the very situation we most fear. This in turn provides evidence that justifies them further, causing them to become even more entrenched.

A woman whose father committed suicide had a strong fear of being abandoned by men. So she would never let a man get too close to her. She would tell herself, "Men cannot be trusted to be there for you. Needing them just sets you up for grief (like I felt when my father died)." This story became a life script that also gave her an identity: "I don't need anyone." Yet stifling her need for closeness made her come across in a tight, held-back way. Since this kept men from feeling close to her, they invariably wound up leaving her. Thus the story she told herself kept recreating her primal abandonment drama. In believing that her story *was* reality, she was blind to how it *created* her reality.

Until we bring consciousness to bear on what we are doing, we will continually recreate our childhood tragedies throughout our lives. The unresolved issues *within* us will continually get acted out as conflicts *between* us and our intimate partners.

PROJECTING AND POLARIZING

As the first blush of falling in love wears off, two partners' scripts increasingly take over and influence their perceptions of each other. Unconsciously assigning each other roles in their inner dramas, they project their hopes and fears, co-creating a distorted reality that can be destructive to them both.

Moreover, people often choose a partner with a script that is the mirror reversal of their own. Thus a person with a fear of engulfment will pair up with someone who has a fear of abandonment. David and Jan were such a couple. Whenever his fear came up, he would create distance. This in turn would bring up her fear, which would make her grab at him, further activating his fear of engulfment. "Pressing each other's buttons" in this way, they became polarized in mutually antagonistic positions that threatened to drive them apart.[3]

Jan's father had been emotionally distant, and this had made her distrustful that a man could ever be there for her. Thus she regarded David's need for solitude and "his own space" as a constant threat. She was always wary that David might be on the verge of leaving her, and would repeatedly seek proof that he really loved her. David, on the other hand, became suspicious whenever women expressed their affection too ardently or demanded his in return. His father had been a busy executive who had little time for his family; as a result, David's mother had turned to her son to fill her emotional needs. Feeling overwhelmed by his mother's needs, and lacking protection from his father, David had learned to protect himself by keeping a safe distance from her.

So when Jan approached him out of her abandonment panic, he became claustrophobic and went into an engulfment panic. He could not understand Jan's urgency unless she was, like his mother, out to eat him alive. And Jan could not understand why he would be so unwilling to give her what she needed unless he was, like her father, distant, punishing, and cold. Their fights, underneath all their convoluted tangles, had a single theme: (Jan) "You're abandoning me." (David) "No, you're being demanding and attacking." (Jan) "No, you're abandoning me." (David) "No, you're engulfing me." Both of them were dreaming up a similar story: that the one they loved was also their oppressor. In reality, neither of them fit this role. Yet insofar as these stories colored their perceptions, Jan and David could not see each other clearly or perceive what was going on between them.

To avoid feeling the pain of old wounds from childhood, each of us has gone unconscious or asleep in certain parts of ourselves. Out of this sleep, we dream up fearful imaginings about our intimate partner. In disowning parts of ourselves, we make them *other*, projecting them outside ourselves and over-reacting to them when we see them there. Most serious relation-ship conflicts are fueled by this kind of projection.[4]

Thus when my partner expresses something I fear in my-self, I may recoil in an exaggerated way. If I am afraid of my anger, hers feels overwhelming. If I can't stand my need, hers makes me feel claustrophobic. I react to my partner's anger or need by pushing her away because I am afraid to experience these feelings myself. Consequently, my inner struggle against unwanted parts of myself turns into an outer struggle with her.

Yet try as we may to ignore parts of ourselves, our larger intelligence wants us to recognize them, so that we can live more fully by having access to the whole of our experience. Thus it was no accident that Jan and David had chosen each other. *Their larger intelligence drew them together because they could help each other heal old wounds and recover important missing pieces of themselves.* Yet this healing could not occur as long as they related to their projections unconsciously—actually seeing each other as the *source* of their fear and reacting in exaggerated ways.

Couples in this kind of struggle have a choice. They can insist that their fearful imaginings are reality, in which case these projections will become solid barriers between them. Or else they can bring awareness to their exaggerated reactions, and use these projections as signposts to point to disowned parts of themselves they need to integrate. When a couple can use their conflict to develop this kind of awareness, it can serve them as path, by helping them wake up from their scripts, relate to old needs and fears in new ways, and thus develop a stronger connection.

EMPOWERING OURSELVES IN OUR PLACE OF NEED

Fortunately for their relationship, Jan and David had a deep, passionate connection that they did not want to lose. Since they had also suffered enough from playing out their projections in past relationships, they were ready and determined to work with their conflict in a new way.

The first step in using a relationship conflict as path is to shift our focus away from the heat of the struggle with our partner and explore its source inside ourselves. Any serious relationship struggle can always point us to wounded places inside ourselves that we have turned away from, and that need attention and healing. At the core of such wounds is a painful inner contraction and conflict around some essential need that we have. An "essential" need—such as to love or to be ourselves—is one that comes from our being, our basic desire to live as fully as we can. Thus at the bottom of most serious relationship struggles, underneath all the projection and defensiveness, are essential needs that we are not acknowledging or that we are expressing in distorted ways.

When we express real needs in distorted ways, it is usually because we are under the influence of the accusing critic or the wounded child within us. The critic makes us feel guilty and ashamed of the need, while the hurt child often acts it out in a compulsive, self-defeating way. Often we oscillate between these two extremes. For instance, the wounded child within Jan would become demanding instead of expressing her need for contact straightforwardly. When this drove David away, she would then attack herself for being needy. The more the critic attacks, the more frustrated and furtive the child becomes. And this leads to further fruitless acting out.

To break out of this cycle, we need to empower ourselves by establishing a straightforward, adult relationship with our needs, so that neither the critic nor the wounded child remains in charge. Then we will no longer have to apologize or fight for them. We can begin to express them in clear and simple terms—"I need . . ." "I feel . . ."—a more effective form of communication that usually evokes a positive response from others.

Often we do not know what the real needs underlying a conflict with our partner are, so well have we hidden them from ourselves. Yet we can always bring them to light by paying attention to the pain or fear that the conflict stirs up in us. By "taking our seat" on the edge of our pain, inquiring gently into it, and opening to it, we will eventually come to a sore or frightened place inside: an old wound from childhood. At the core of this wound we will find a genuine need, which we have felt so conflicted about that we have hardly ever recognized or expressed it directly. Usually when it arises in a relationship, we contract—closing down or becoming angry with our partner. Yet if we can make a friendly space for this need, we will find a basic intelligence in it; and this will enable us to trust it and express it more straightforwardly.

In his conflict with Jan, David was in pain about feeling engulfed by her need for loving contact. When he opened to this pain, it connected him with a deep wound from his past: his conflicted feelings about needing to be an individual in his own right. Although he would blame Jan for not letting him have his own space, the truth was that he did not really feel entitled to it. This was because of his guilt about having to push away his mother in order to be himself. Out of this guilt, David had developed critic stories that led him to believe that his need to be himself was somehow wrong, bad, or impossible.

The first step in empowering ourselves in our wounded

places often involves cutting through the critic stories that deflect our attention from our core wound and the essential need hidden within it. In David's case, the critic would tell him, "Why do you always have to prove you're separate? What's the matter with you? You're just afraid of love." Thus whenever he felt Jan's need for contact, he fell into an emotional "bog," a complex tangle of conflicting feelings: helplessness, then contraction, self-critical blame, followed by guilt, leading to his typical final reaction, "Let me out of here."

Identifying and setting aside the critic helped David open to his core wound and his genuine needs—which his critic usually kept him from experiencing. Then he could begin to make friends with his need to have his own space. He discovered that this need contained a wisdom of its own—about the importance of maintaining his integrity in a relationship, finding nourishment in his own being, and not sacrificing any of that just to make another person happy. In honoring the intelligence in his need, he found a power spot: here he could be fully himself, without having to depend on anyone else for fulfillment.

Having found his seat, David no longer needed his old story that "Women are out to eat you alive." Instead of having to fight for space by pushing Jan away, he could express his need for space more simply and directly. Since this made him more emotionally present, Jan no longer felt so threatened.

In a similar way, by exploring the pain she felt in chasing after David, Jan contacted her old wound—her conflicted feelings about needing love. Because she had felt so unfulfilled as a child, part of her had come to believe that she was unworthy of love. Before she could make friends with her need for loving contact, Jan too had to become aware of her critic, who said, "You're so needy—what's wrong with you?" Her usual response to this voice was to collapse and lose her seat—which only made her feel more powerless and needy. This was *her* bog. Through opening to her core wound and learning to face down her critic, she developed the courage to acknowledge her need for love more straightforwardly.

Befriending her need allowed Jan to find her power and

appreciate herself in a new way. She began to realize that the openheartedness in her desire for loving contact was a real strength, rather than a weakness. When she could finally express her desire for closeness simply and directly, David no longer felt so threatened and could be more responsive.

As they made friends with their needs, Jan and David no longer felt compelled to project their fears. No longer seeing each other as oppressors, they could begin to communicate what they were actually experiencing in their conflicts. When Jan could simply say, "I'm feeling abandoned and scared right now," David became less defensive. And when he could say, "I'm feeling overwhelmed and put on the spot," this disarmed her. They also found some humor in the situation by making up names for their respective "bogs," and this gave them a friendly way of reminding each other when they were slipping into an abandonment or engulfment panic.

ALONE TOGETHER

Needs always come in pairs—to be alone, to be together; to talk about problems, to set problems aside; to play, to work. So when we empower ourselves in relation to a need we have felt badly about, this frees us to recognize and honor the complementary need, which our partner has usually been representing in our conflicts. And this helps heal the polarization that has developed between us.

This kind of healing is especially important when a couple is at war over the core issue in a relationship—how to negotiate the basic poles of separateness and togetherness. We all have some longing to join and connect with others, as well as a taste for solitude, individual freedom, and space. Only by acknowledging both these sides can we resolve our childhood dramas, develop more healthy relationships, and become more whole.

Yet living with an intimate partner while also remaining true to ourselves is a difficult edge. On one hand, a couple cannot remain in a perpetual state of togetherness. Because two lovers are always separate people, each with his or her own experiences, temperaments, preferences, rhythms, and path, they can never realize absolute union in any conclusive, uninterrupted way. Trying to feel secure by establishing an identity as a "we" only creates addiction and inner impoverishment. It causes us to neglect the deep, silent springs of vitality inside us and the simple truth of our experience, which often emerges most powerfully in moments when we are not involved in "relating" at all. No matter how close to another person we may be, part of us is radically and forever alone and, in its own way, wild and free. If we use a relationship to deny this, it can only be superficial or distorted, for it will not be aligned with reality.

On the other hand, if we deny or suppress our need for contact, we also distort our nature. There is no such thing as a totally independent individual. A vast network of relationship connects us to other people and to the cosmos as a whole. Love warms us and opens us to life. Therefore, to be fully ourselves we also need to be warmly engaged with others.

The final healing of the rift between Jan and David happened as they came to recognize, through working on themselves, that both these needs—to be strong individuals and to be close to each other—belonged equally to each of them. As she came to accept her need for love, Jan discovered why it had always been so hard to feel: It brought up her terror of being left alone. She had hated her aloneness as a child because it was associated with deprivation, which had felt like a threat to her survival. By relating to her inner child in a caring way and educating her to the present situation—that being alone was no longer a threat to her survival—Jan loosened the hold that her old abandonment stories had on her.

Then, instead of looking to David to save her from being alone, Jan became more interested in finding out who *she* was. She discovered that her aloneness was not a deficiency, and that honoring it only enriched her connection with David. She even started to enjoy setting aside solitary time in which to explore her own connection with life. She began to appreciate that, as Thomas Merton once said, "In solitude we remain face to face with the naked being of things." In reflecting on this period in her life, Jan wrote, "An essential step in developing my strength and overcoming my fear of loss came when I accepted my aloneness and discovered a deep sense of relatedness to the earth, to trees, water, the dark of night, and the seasons of the year . . ."

Similarly, when David could finally take the space he needed in their relationship without guilt, he no longer needed to hold on to his old engulfment stories. This also allowed him to reconnect with all his buried sorrow and grief about having had to close his heart to his mother so many years before. When he realized how he had been living with a contracted heart all his life, he started to feel a new desire: to radiate his love more freely and magnanimously, without having to hold back. He began to feel his own need for contact and enjoy pursuing Jan when she was taking *her* space. As Jan began to explore and enjoy her aloneness, he also got to feel what it was like to be on the other side. One day, when he began worrying that *she* might not need *him* anymore, he knew that something new was really happening!

Now that David no longer had to assert his separateness defiantly, and Jan no longer regarded it as a threat, they could join together on a new basis, honoring themselves and each other more fully as individuals. A new freedom and space entered their relationship. This period of exploring and reclaiming the "other" side of themselves marked an important stage in their development, both as individuals and as a couple.

Through their struggles Jan and David had learned a powerful, essential lesson: *that relationship, rather than being just a form of togetherness, is a ceaseless flowing back and forth between joining and separating.* Just as the moon begins to wane at the peak of its fullness and the tide ebbs at the height of its flux, so after moments of intense connecting two partners naturally begin to fall back into their aloneness. And in moments when they feel most separate, a desire is born to come together again. The health of a relationship depends on both partners being able to move freely back and forth between these two poles.

This is a key discovery for every relationship. We often imagine that having our own space in a relationship is the opposite of being intimate. Yet actually the reverse is true: *Space is what allows intimacy to happen.* It enables two people to meet and touch freshly, to "see each other whole and against a wide sky," as Rilke put it. Rilke's lover, Lou Andreas-Salome, concurred when she wrote, "Two are at one only when they remain two." The electricity in a couple's erotic connection flows most freely when they are not entangled, but rather feel themselves as two distinct, separate poles, man and woman.

Whenever one partner identifies with togetherness or separateness as an end in itself, this will only set up a struggle with the other partner, who, consciously or not, will feel compelled to compensate for this unbalanced position. Yet if we can see these struggles as helping us learn to balance different sides of ourselves, we can regard them more cheerfully—not as acts of war, but as steps in learning to dance.

In this way, we can learn to use every obstacle we meet on the path of relationship as part of the path itself. Our conflicts with our partner help us identify and contact essential missing pieces of ourselves. In making friends with these parts of ourselves, we free up a wider range of our powers and possibilities. We begin to fill out, to soften and expand, and this allows love to flow through us more freely and unobstructedly.

10

Developing Larger Vision

ALL OF LOVE'S POWER AND CREATIVITY arises out of the play of differences. Yet when these differences harden into oppositions, they arouse fear and antagonism, which can tear apart the very fabric of a relationship. The most fundamental difference in a relationship is between "self" and "other." Whenever this difference becomes solidified into "for" and "against" positions— "self" is right and "other" is wrong—the dance of relationship grinds to a halt and turns into a tug of war. When the mind hardens into an oppositional stance, we lose flexibility and fluidity—which are our greatest resources in handling conflict. If we are to use relationship difficulties as opportunities for growth instead of being defeated by them, we must be able to free ourselves from the grip of "oppositional mind."

In the martial arts, developing a fluid awareness that does not freeze into opposition is often a matter of life and death. If the samurai's mind "stops" for a moment to oppose what is happening—his opponent's lunge toward him or his opponent's sword as it falls through the air—this may endanger his life. It slows him down and prevents him from making necessary split-second changes and adjustments. For this reason, many samurai warriors in ancient Japan studied Zen meditation. As a practice of freeing attention from fixating on any thought, perception, or attitude, meditation taught the samurai how to develop a more flexible, panoramic awareness.

Similarly, to move more fluidly with the shifting challenges of an intimate relationship, we need to develop a wider-angle vision that does not become stuck in opposition. This requires stepping out of habitual mind-sets—what we already know or believe—so that we can take a fresh look at what is going on. Then two partners can find a higher ground they both can share—a larger, panoramic perspective on what is happening between them, beyond their conflicting, egocentric points of view.

MIRRORING

One simple yet effective way to expand our normally narrow field of vision is by regarding whatever is happening in a relationship as a mirror that can reflect something important back to us about ourselves. The basic principle is simple: Two partners are like a pair of multifaceted mirrors, and their interaction picks up and reflects sides of each other that they might not otherwise see as clearly. Moreover, the way we relate to others always reflects the way we relate to parts of ourselves. We could modify the old alchemical motto—"As above, so below"—to express this fundamental truth in all human interactions: "As without, so within." The dramas we enact in relationships are the dramas we carry inside us. The qualities we seek in a partner are the qualities we also need to find within ourselves. And what we reject in others points to parts of ourselves that we also do not accept.

Regarding relationship as a mirror can help expand our awareness of what is happening in our interactions. We can ask of any dynamic that is happening or of any irritation we feel toward our partner, "What is this mirroring in me? What is this forcing me to look at in myself?" Instead of focusing on what the other person is doing wrong, we can then begin to see where *we* need to grow. In this way, we can use whatever frustrations or limitations we come up against in a relationship as part of our path.

It is easy to focus on what is wrong with our partner or with the relationship. What is usually much harder to see is how we ourselves always help create whatever problem exists—if only through how we perceive and react to what is going on. In fact, *every* difficulty in a relationship is co-created. It is much harder to change our partner or "fix" the relationship than it is to work on how we contribute to the difficulty. Surprisingly, when we work on ourselves, the relationship usually starts improving as well.

This doesn't mean that we should always take everything on ourselves, while completely overlooking the ways we would like our partner to change. That would be going to the other extreme. Rather, the purpose of regarding relationship as a mirror is to reverse our usual oppositional mind-set of focusing exclusively on what our partner is doing, while ignoring how we are both co-creating the situation.

As an example of how mirroring can work, consider the situation of a talented young doctor who complained that his wife did not appreciate or support him. No matter how much he tried to win her favor, she would never praise him. Yet why did he have such a need for her praise? What was this mirroring in him? When he explored this, he realized that he felt like a child, rather than a powerful man, in her company. Instead of taking care of himself, he expected her to make him feel okay. Seeing what *he* was doing allowed him to shift gears, to assert and appreciate himself more in the relationship instead of seeking her approval. When he did this, she suddenly started to express her admiration and appreciation for the first time. She had not deliberately made this change. It was her spontaneous response to a different quality of energy happening between them as the result of his work on himself.

Another example: A woman who always wound up with alcoholic men would struggle, with little success, to reform them by trying to give them faith in themselves. Her preoccupation with *their* problems kept her from paying attention to what this unsatisfactory situation pointed to in herself. She too lacked self-esteem. The motivation behind her crusade to rescue these men was her own need to feel worthwhile. When she began to address this lack of confidence in herself, she no longer needed to save alcoholic men.

Mirroring happens not only between intimate partners, but in any relationship where two people are working closely. For example, in my early days as a psychotherapist, when clients resisted change, I would try out different strategies to overcome their resistance—which invariably led nowhere. When I instead used clients' resistance as a mirror, I saw that I *was resisting their resistance.* This led to a curious but extremely helpful discovery: Often the most useful thing to do in such situations was to work on my own resistance and give clients more space to go through whatever they needed to. Then they had less need to resist me or the work!

One woman I worked with often complained that "men are not emotionally available." Maybe this is true, maybe not. But her story about men put her in conflict with them from the start. When she went out on a date, she would immediately try to get the man to be more open to her, which only made him want to pull away instead. How could she use mirroring to help clarify the situation? I held the mirror up to her by asking, "The main problem you see in relationships is men's emotional unavailability. Is there any part of *you* that is unavailable?" Since my suggestion threatened her righteous position, she refused to consider this at first, firmly replying, "No." So I asked her, "Not even a little bit? Not even one percent of you?" As she looked at this further, she began to discover ways in which she was indeed keeping herself distant. She had a deep, unacknowledged rage against men, as well as a fear of being mistreated by them. This led her to isolate certain parts of herself from a relationship in order to feel safe. Choosing unavailable men allowed her to focus on their problems instead of having to face her own unavailability.

I also asked the man she was seeing to consider his complaint about her as a mirror: "The main problem you see in this relationship is that she is run by her feelings. Is there any way in which your feelings run you?" At first he rejected this invitation to look at himself like this because it threatened his story about himself as cool, calm, and collected. Eventually he came to see that he avoided discussing feelings because he was afraid of where that might lead. His partner's greater facility in this area also intimidated him. So in refusing to talk about his feelings with her, he too was run by his feelings—of fear. When he looked in the mirror instead of blaming his partner, he had a path and somewhere to go: He needed to look at what he was so afraid of and how he let his fear control him.

Recognizing that they each had the very problems that they were blaming their partner for lessened this couple's opposition. It provided some common ground for working with their differences, resulting in a greater spirit of friendliness. And it pointed to areas in themselves that needed attention if their relationship was to keep growing.

So whenever we feel stuck or confused about a particular relationship or about relationships as a whole, we can often find a way forward by treating the problem as a mirror—of some unfinished business inside us that we have not yet clearly seen. Here are some briefer examples that illustrate how relationship problems mirror inner blind spots:

1. A woman is angry with men because they always criticize her and withhold their love. She does not see that this is also how she treats herself: She withholds love from herself by allying with her inner critic. She chooses men who are not there for her because this is a familiar situation for her—she is not there for herself. Until she works on this in herself, her relationships will not go very far.

2. A man who considers himself impeccable about keeping his word and being reliable finds women untrustworthy. He always winds up with "unreliable" women because he is attracted to their vivaciousness and spontaneity, qualities that his stern dedication to being steady and reliable has eclipsed in himself. Nevertheless, his attraction to such women is a sign that he is trying to come into relationship with these exiled qualities

in himself. Instead of engaging in a crusade to make women more reliable, he needs to work on freeing up his own spontaneity.

3. A sweet young man always winds up with aggressive women who hurt him. This situation reflects his need to get in touch with his own aggression, which hides behind his ever-present smile. It is no accident that he regards women as bitchy and pushy. His oversensitivity to these qualities in women reflects his uneasiness about being assertive himself. He fears women's rage because he fears his own denied anger. His attraction to powerful women reflects his need to find his own power.

4. A playful, lighthearted woman, after many years of marriage, is having a hard time accepting her husband's seriousness and intensity. Her partner is not really the problem, however. She has disowned her own darker side, which she has conveniently let him play out all these years. Her present dissatisfaction indicates that letting him express that side of her no longer works for her. She needs to get to know her own darkness.

5. A man who loves to save damsels in distress invariably winds up being left by them after he rescues them from their difficulties. What does this situation reflect? There is a part of himself that needs to be "saved": his own inner femininity, his softness and sensitivity, which he denies. Being out of touch with it makes him brittle and constricted. So when the women he saves begin to blossom, they do not find their newfound fullness reflected in him, and must go elsewhere.

FOURFOLD TRUTH

Another way to cultivate larger vision and overcome oppositional mind is by recognizing how truth and distortion are always operating on both sides of any relationship conflict. This is because we all embody a mixture of wisdom and karmic entanglements, sanity and neurosis. Therefore we rarely speak with a single tongue of unalloyed clarity and truth. On one hand, our unconditioned being—our "wisdom mind" or "wisdom heart"—naturally wants to connect with things as they are. In this sensitivity and responsiveness to reality lie our basic sanity and goodness. Yet at the same time, our conditioned personality finds security through maintaining and defending its habitual *version* of reality. Our need to convince ourselves that the way we see things is the "Truth" may be so strong that we are often willing to harm a relationship just to prove that we are "right."

Yet though our blind spots, projections, hopes, and fears inevitably introduce distortions into our relationships, the saving grace is that something genuine inside us is always trying to shine through. Even though when I fall in love, I distort the situation by projecting my own unrecognized power and radiance onto my beloved, I am also perceiving her real beauty at the same time. And I am trying, in a roundabout way, to connect with my larger being.

Similarly, no matter how crazy my partner and I become in our fights with each other, there is usually some kernel of truth in what each of us is trying to express. Yet when I set myself in opposition to her, trying to prove myself right and her wrong, I can see only my own truth and her distortions. She does the same with me. Yet we *are* both expressing some truth. The problem is that we do not also see our own distortions. As a result, we hold things against each other, and our opposition hardens.

For example, a man who needs more space in a relationship may distort this truth by projecting his fears of his mother onto his partner and thus resenting her need for closeness. This will make it hard for her to hear and appreciate his truth because she will feel compelled to show him that he is wrong.

Her truth is that she wants him to engage with her more fully. Yet she may express this need in a distorted way, through pressuring or blaming him. This only makes it harder for him to hear, much less appreciate, her need for closeness.

One way a couple can work with such a deadlock is through recognizing fourfold truth: that each of their sides has both a genuine and a distorted component. In encouraging a couple to do this, I ask them each to state their truth simply, and follow this by acknowledging to each other the distorted way it has been coming across. When one partner can openly acknowledge his distortions to the other and listen to her truth in turn, her cause for resentment and opposition starts to fall away. She no longer has to fight to get him to see her side. As the issue of who is right and who is wrong loses importance, they can begin to really hear each other for a change.

Unfortunately, it is not always easy to distinguish what is genuine in our experience from what is distorted. That is where an awareness practice such as mindfulness meditation or present-centered psychotherapy can be particularly useful. These disciplines slow down the busy mind. By sharpening awareness and discernment, they can help us separate our immediate experience from our stories. They teach us how to create a friendly, unbiased space, free from blame, in which we can distinguish simple truths from the paranoid imaginings of oppositional mind.

To clear up the distortions that accumulate and clog the flow of love in a relationship, we may want to create this kind of friendly listening space with our partner whenever we become locked into serious opposition. I have found that it is often helpful to deliberately set aside time with my partner—an hour, a day, or a weekend—to articulate our different truths and untangle our distortions. This works best if we begin by mutually affirming our willingness to listen to each other and acknowledge our distortions, and our intention not to make each other wrong or freeze into defensive reactions. Then each of us can take turns airing what needs to be said, while the other listens and simply repeats back the main points. After that, the listening partner can respond. We continue to go back and forth like that until we each feel that the other has really heard us. As our distortions come to light, we may feel and express genuine remorse about how we have hurt each other. Sharing this also helps bring us closer again.

TRUSTING THE RELATIONSHIP AS
A TEACHER

Often two partners become locked in opposition not just to each other, but to the whole situation they are in. When this happens, an extremely helpful way to develop larger vision and overcome oppositional mind is by recognizing whatever is happening between them as a teacher.

When two people create a path together, it is as though their individual intelligence and wisdom join together in a synergistic way, acting as a larger, guiding force that can show them each where they most need to grow. As an expression of life's basic movement toward greater wholeness working in and through their relationship, this "couple intelligence" can be an accurate and trustworthy guide. When two partners appreciate that their connection invariably points them in the direction of growth, they can begin to regard *any* situation that comes up in their relationship as a teacher.

One way that such "couple intelligence" works is through a natural balancing process. Anything that one partner ignores, the other will feel a greater need to emphasize. Whatever quality of being I deny, such as power, softness, or playfulness, my partner will find herself feeling an urge to express more strongly. Just as when I deny my anger, my stomach may act it out for me in the form of indigestion, so my partner may enact it in the form of unreasonable rages. All I want is peace and quiet, while she is suddenly angry about every little thing! Regarding the relationship as a teacher means that I can trust that what is happening between us contains a certain intelligence. So I can step back and ask myself, "She is always angry these days—what is this trying to teach me?" If I do this, I will find that this situation contains an important message for me.

Here are some more examples of how a couple can use what is going on in their interaction as a teacher:

One couple I know were both feeling restless after being together for three years. At first, they were tempted to make up scare stories such as, "Maybe our relationship is over." If they kept going in that direction, their stories would have become self-fulfilling prophecies. Instead, they took a different tack, regarding their restlessness as a teacher. This helped them to see how they had each been using their relationship to make things safe and to avoid branching out into new areas of personal development. The restlessness that at first seemed like such a threat to their relationship was pointing to certain unrealized potentials, which they had been trying to ignore.

Another couple found themselves going through a period of intense fighting in their second year of being together, and did not know what to make of it. They both imagined that their relationship was about to self-destruct. Yet when they looked for the intelligence in their fighting, they found that it was a sign that they were going deeper with each other than they had ever gone before with anyone else. Their fights were expressing deep-seated fears that needed to be recognized and dealt with. When they saw this, they could address their fears more directly. This relieved the panic that something was desperately wrong with their relationship and helped them keep moving forward.

A third couple became upset when their sexual desire seemed to disappear for a long stretch of time. It was easy to imagine that their passion for each other had finally exhausted itself. Yet when they looked more closely at the situation, they found that they were both yearning for a deeper sexual connection with each other. It was as though some larger intelligence in them wanted their old routine, predictable sexual patterns to wither away, so that something new could emerge. Although they were not sure what this new kind of sexuality would be like, they found their way by setting aside time to be with each other in a sensual way, without any agenda, and paying attention to how their energies wanted to connect.

At times a couple's larger intelligence may be a firm taskmaster, forcing them to face unpleasant truths and learn lessons they would rather avoid. It may be urging them in new directions, despite their reluctance to go there. ("This is too much. I didn't get involved in a relationship in order to deal with *this*.")

Yet this "couple intelligence" can be trusted because its aim is greater wholeness and vitality.

If a couple does not respond to what their interaction is prodding them to learn, the lesson will usually keep coming back in harsher, more forceful ways until it finally commands their attention. Consider the case of one couple who refused to regard what was happening in their marriage as a teacher. After eight years together, they began to notice an increasing sense of emptiness and distance between them. This brought up feelings of loneliness and fear of loss, which neither of them wanted to face. So, instead of consciously exploring the emptiness they felt and using it as a guide to help them work on things between them, they tried to fill it up by taking other lovers. This caused their marriage to fall apart, but so slowly and painfully that they each lost their lovers as well. Then they each had to face their emptiness in a much more painful way. It would have been wiser to look for the intelligence in the emptiness they were feeling, align themselves with it, and learn from it. This would have allowed them to find the direction of growth contained in their impasse.

Regarding the situations that crop up in relationships as teachers can help us avoid fighting with them, which only wastes energy. Instead, as in the dance of aikido, we can learn to move *with* whatever is happening and use it to further our unfolding.

PRACTICING BEGINNER'S MIND

To step out of oppositional mind and develop larger vision on the spot, we must put aside our stories about what is going on, so that we can take a fresh look at whatever situation we are in. When we do this, we come back to the present moment, which is as sharp and thin as a razor's edge. This always involves a slight jolt, which wakes us up. These little moments of waking up are pulsing with uncertainty. At such moments the most honest statement we can make about how to proceed is, *"I don't know."* How could I know? I just arrived here.

For some, admitting that they do not know is a sign of weakness. Yet for the warrior of the heart, who honors the great unknown surrounding him on all sides, acknowledging the truth of not-knowing is like a cool breeze. It clears away the clouds of the busy mind, allowing a fresh and precise response to what is happening in the present moment. To keep refreshing our perception in this way is to practice *beginner's mind.* When we can face what is happening without relying on old stories or beliefs to interpret it, we invite our larger intelligence, free of attachment to fixed views, to guide us.

When a businessman I know returned home from a month-long trip, he and his wife had a hard time finding common ground again. Their first reaction to each other was "Who are you?" for they had been having very different experiences in their time apart, and were in very different places. This disconcerted them, bringing up fear and uncertainty about their relationship. At such times, the mind's tendency is to jump to some conclusion. So each of them could feel the temptation to concoct a story to explain what was going on—"Something has happened," "Things are not the same between us," "We are drifting apart." Yet they managed to resist this temptation, agreeing, "Let's just let this gap be there for now. Let's not try to fix it or make up any stories about it." Then, as they naturally began to reconnect over the next few days, they found their interaction newly vibrant and alive because they had so much to tell each other about the different things they had experienced. They were heartened to find that they could trust their love to recreate itself, without deliberately trying to make it happen.

This couple could more readily proceed in this way because they had learned, after going through many changes together, that a relationship can only renew itself by shedding its old skins. Early in their marriage they had become firmly entrenched in classic co-dependent positions: He was the big, strong man who took care of their relations with the world, while she was the doting female who took care of him at home. When they both finally rebelled against the burdens of this arrangement, their relationship went through a major crisis. What would bind them together if they no longer needed each other to fill these old co-dependent roles? Should they move forward and risk losing everything, or should they stay stuck where they were and feel miserable?

This kind of crisis happens in every relationship, often many times, for the initial ways in which two people fit together are usually shaped by old childhood scripts that they must eventually leave behind. Also, the way two people adapt to each other one year may no longer be appropriate the next, once they have grown in new ways. Yet moving beyond our old dependencies and adaptations requires a scary leap into the unknown. Often we are unsure of just what is happening, or whether our relationship can survive such major changes.

This is when practicing beginner's mind—not holding on to any fixed idea about how things are supposed to be—becomes essential. If my partner and I let go of our old structures, how will we then relate to each other? We cannot know that in advance. What we do know is that some larger urge is tugging at us and that if we ignore it, we run the risk of stagnation and degeneration.

One couple who had been married for twenty-five years came for counseling after the wife seriously began to question whether they should stay together any longer. Underneath all their specific dissatisfactions, it soon became apparent that they were not making any real contact with each other. Their interactions consisted mainly of talking *at* each other—lecturing each other, musing, telling stories, philosophizing, criticizing—instead of ever being present, simply sharing the moment together. This lack of satisfying contact was impoverishing their relationship more than anything else.

Bringing this to their attention, I asked them just to be present with each other on the spot, without going into their usual routines. This made them both uncomfortable because it meant *not knowing what to do.* Each time they would go off into lecturing or talking at each other in broad, general terms, I would ask them to come back and see what it was like to stay in contact without knowing what to do. This forced them to give up playing it safe. At first they felt helpless, then frightened, then angry, then discouraged and sad.

After going through all these reactions, this couple eventually began to see the humor in their situation: Despite twenty-five years of relating, they still did not know how to relate. When they let themselves appreciate this, it felt as though they were meeting for the first time, and a new freshness and excitement started entering their contact. From that point on, this couple had a path.

If a couple is willing to let the patterns their relationship has settled into die, it can keep being reborn. And they may find their connection deepening with every death and rebirth, taking on a further sense of adventure as it prods them to keep moving in new directions. However, two people's egos often collude to cover up these crucial moments of flux and transition. They may blame each other for the changes that are happening. Or they may scramble to put on their old masks, trying to find security in their familiar views of one another: "He needs me because I am warm and he is cold," "She needs me to tell her what to do," "He's fragile, so I can't be honest with him," "Without me, she'll never get it together."

Of course, two people *do* come to know each other's habits and patterns quite intimately, and there is always truth in these perceptions. They distort things, however, when they let such stories substitute for perceiving each other freshly. In assuming that they know each other fully, they create predictable routines that constrict the larger life energy flowing between them.

So if I put all my stories aside and simply look into my beloved's eyes, what do I see? Who is she? I find nothing I can readily grasp—only an open space stretching deep into the unknown. Looking into her eyes makes me realize the shocking truth of the matter—I don't *really* know who she is at all. I may know her patterns—how she thinks and reacts to things—but does that mean that I really know who she is? If I am completely truthful as our eyes meet, I can only say, "Hello. Who are you? For that matter, who am I?" In such moments of beginner's mind, all my investments in who I am and who she is fall away.

Such moments are like waking up in the morning and suddenly not knowing for an instant who we are or what we are doing here. This can be so abrupt and shocking that we quickly brush it aside. It may cause us to freeze in panic, or scurry to find some familiar story or habit to assure ourselves that we are the same old person we always thought we were. Yet such moments can also be a healthy, invigorating reminder that we have a new chance at life each day. No matter how much we think we know, it is only a tiny fraction of all that we don't know. Who we are is not who we have been. The truth is that we can never fully know who we are, where we come from, or where we are ultimately going. Recognizing this keeps us honest and awake. It allows us to keep unfolding in new directions.

Couples often ask, "How can we keep our love alive and growing after so many years together?" Individuals wonder, "How can I keep my freedom and still be in a committed relationship?" Cultivating a taste for the unknown—which opens up when we let our stories go and face our partner freshly—is the essential key to maintaining freedom in a relationship and keeping love alive. The truth is that two people can never completely penetrate the mystery of their connection and know what it is. Realizing that our most intimate relationship is never just what we thought dissolves opposition and brings renewal. If two people can face each other in a spirit of beginner's mind, they will discover that their connection can continually expand beyond domestic familiarity, to include a larger sense of space and mystery.

PART III

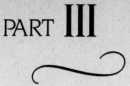

Sacred Path

11

Natural Sacredness

> When you experience your wisdom and the power
> of things as they are, together, as one, then you
> have access to tremendous vision and power in the
> world. You find that you are inherently connected
> to your own being. That is discovering magic.
>
> CHÖGYAM TRUNGPA

LOVE AS A PERSONAL PATH involves plowing the coarse and rocky ground of ego, breaking up the hardened places inside us, refining and enriching this soil so that life can grow more abundantly in us. Then, having begun to cultivate our earth, we can start to grow in the direction of the open sky. Sacred path involves taking this further step: opening more fully to the vastness of our being, connecting directly with the larger energies moving in and through our relationships, and bringing these more fully into our daily life.

DISCOVERING SACRED VISION

I do not use the term *sacred* here in any conventional religious sense. Nor do I mean to suggest that sacredness descends from something "on high"—a deity or heavenly paradise existing up above us somewhere. Such a view tends to split reality into two disjointed parts: a profane or degraded earth below and a pure, holy heaven on high. We do not have to regard sacredness as something added onto life through special activities or beliefs. Nor do we have to "get religion" or be "born again" in some dramatic way to discover it.

Life has its own natural sacredness, which shines through most brightly *when we get out of the way*—when we set aside old stories and beliefs that contribute to oppositional mind-sets, pitting "self" against the world as "other." In those moments when we can step outside the struggle between self and other, and simply open ourselves to what is, we begin to perceive the natural, sacred order—of earth and sky, life and death, mind, heart, and body—behind all the seeming chaos of the world. When "the doors of perception are cleansed" in this way, we can appreciate the magnificence of the whole play of reality, in which self and other are but provisional, shifting points of view.

Human existence is sacred as well because our intelligence is naturally attuned, deep within, to the power and magic of the natural order, the pattern that connects heaven and earth. We intuitively know what is wholesome and life-promoting, and can distinguish that from what is corrupt and life-negating. When we appreciate the simple beauty and power at work in all of creation, and choose to live in alignment with that larger vision, we tap into our basic human wisdom. And we discover sacred vision.

Pretechnological cultures, living close to the earth, always recognized the basic human need to connect with life's larger energies. This kind of attunement was the sacred pivot point of an individual's life, around which lesser worldly concerns revolved. For the American Indian, the most ordinary activities— whether hunting an animal, eating a meal, teaching a child, sitting down with friends, or simply marking the passage of time and the seasons—were all opportunities to appreciate the sacredness of life.

Even the famous "sitting bull" posture expresses a sacred attitude. By aligning the body with heaven and earth, this universal meditation posture reveals how to approach our lives and relationships in an expansive, yet fully grounded way. In taking our seat on the earth—slowing down and simply being present—we tap into *profundity,* the nourishing depth of our being. When we come from this ground of well-being, oppositional struggles—either fighting with or clinging to others in order to make ourselves feel better—fall away. And in facing forward into the larger space before us, we tap into *vastness,* the greater possibilities within us that lead us to venture beyond where we have already been.

Unfortunately, our technological society, in pursuing the conquest of nature, has disrupted our natural connectedness with these elemental powers moving within us. Being cut off from the profundity of earth and the vastness of heaven in our lives leaves us with an unnameable sense of deprivation and hunger, prey to what often seem to be strange, reckless urges to connect with something meaningful and intense. Husbands and wives suddenly leave their marriages after thirty years, in search of a nameless fulfillment. Adolescents become involved with drugs, sometimes destroying their lives in search of something that can engage them intensely. People of all ages become susceptible to extremist cults that promise to fill the vacuum they feel inside.

Similarly, we may turn to intimate relationships to fill our hunger for the sacred. However, our need to experience awe and devotion in the face of all that is greater than ourselves may cause us to inflate romantic love and regard it as a form of salvation. And this only leads to greater despair and emptiness when we eventually wake up from this delusion. Nonetheless our confused attempts to use romance to satisfy all our spiritual yearnings do point to an underlying truth: The love between man and woman can provide powerful glimpses of sacred vision.

Love has sacred power not because it makes us high, allowing us to rise above ordinary life on clouds of blissful glory, but because it helps us relax the struggle between self and other that is at the root of human suffering. Love is profound because it roots us in the earth, shining its light on all the different sides of who we are, including those we would rather not have to look at. The profound question love poses is, "Can you face your life as it is; can you look at all the pain and darkness as well as the power and light in the human soul, and still say yes?" And love is vast because it makes us want to keep growing and expanding without limit. It allows us to use all the garbage we find inside ourselves as compost—to nourish the growth of awareness, courage, and compassion and to enlarge our capacity for relating to life as a whole.

So it is important not to get too starry-eyed when contemplating the spiritual dimension of love. For we can bring love's sacred dimension into everyday life only by respecting and attending to the most simple and mundane details of our relationships. Although sacred vision may be vast and profound, it is also quite ordinary. It is a question of honoring the elemental qualities of things as they are—whether it be the solidity of earth, the heat of passion, the fierceness of anger, or the pain of a broken heart. This is why great spiritual masters irreverently cut through any pompous religiosity on their students' part. "Where is Buddha to be found?" the earnest disciple asks. "The cypress tree in the dooryard," the Zen master replies. Even more pointedly, the master might answer, "The dogshit in the grass." Or simply, "Go scrub the floor." Life's ordinary magic lies right in front of us when we relate fully and directly to things as they are.

As long as we hold to conventional attitudes that allow us to see only one side of a situation at a time, we remain trapped in oppositional mind and lose touch with sacred vision. That is why spiritual teachers often act outrageously, outside the bounds of normal convention: to jar people loose from the habitual mind-set that makes reality appear one-dimensional. Sacred outlook is born in moments when our familiar ways of looking at things start to break down, when we are lifted out of ourselves and freed from "single-eyed vision." At such times we suddenly have a chance to see without filters, to *see life whole, in all its contradictions*—which no thought can ever encompass. Although it may feel painful when our small version of reality breaks open, it is also illuminating, as Job discovered when his world collapsed and God revealed to him the unspeakable vastness of life beyond his worldly concerns.

In this light, the difficult challenges that men and women encounter in joining their energies together are not just personal travails. They are also invitations to open ourselves to the sacred play of the known and the unknown, the seen and the unseen, and to the larger powers born out of intimate contact with the great mysteries of life.

12

In Search of the Genuine, Powerful Male and Female

> If we were men, if we were women, our
> individualities would be lone and a bit mysterious,
> like tarns, and fed with power, male power, female
> power, from underneath, invisibly. And from us the
> streams of desire would flow out in the eternal
> glimmering adventure . . .
>
> D. H. LAWRENCE

FOR THOUSANDS OF YEARS the relations between men and women
have been clouded and distorted by unrealistic fantasies. Projecting our hopes and fears, we have idealized each other as
angels and saviors or maligned each other as monsters and
demons. Rarely have we recognized each other as whole human
beings.

Now, with all the traditional sex roles and stereotypes
breaking down, even *our own* maleness or femaleness, which
used to be taken for granted, has become a matter of uncertainty
and doubt. Yet the current upheaval going on within men and
women also provides a new opportunity—to uncover a more
essential maleness or femaleness concealed beneath our old
conventional roles. The present situation challenges us to dig
deep and ask the most fundamental questions. How can we
bring forth the authentic, powerful male or female energies

from within us? How can we draw on these elemental energies to deepen our sense of who we are and what we have to give each other? How can men and women overcome the oppositional struggles that have plagued them for thousands of years and forge a new kind of creative alliance?

Since there are few sources of external guidance to draw on, we each have to undertake our own individual search to find out what it means to be an authentic, powerful man or woman. This search begins by digging down through conventional notions of manliness or womanliness and considering what is valid for ourselves as individuals. In doing this, we soon discover that masculine qualities do not belong to men alone, any more than feminine qualities belong only to women. Every individual has access to a whole range of masculine and feminine energies. As we cultivate this wider spectrum, our ways of expressing our manhood or womanhood become more flexible and dynamic, rather than stereotypical. This allows us to take a further step: discovering the essential male or female within.

So this search seems to have three main stages:

1. Waking up from socially conditioned sex roles and stereotypes that we have unconsciously acted out.
2. Discovering that both sexes have access to both masculine and feminine energies, and blending and balancing these energies within ourselves.
3. For a man, celebrating the genuine, powerful maleness within him, and for a woman, celebrating her genuine, powerful femaleness. For both sexes, appreciating and living their differences consciously, and using them to help spark each other's growth.

STAGE ONE: RECOGNIZING UNCONSCIOUS SEX ROLES

Our identity as a male or female begins with imitation. From the earliest age, we seek a sexual identity, yet all we can do is imitate the models available to us—parents, older siblings, peers, or images in the media.

People in most cultures through the ages have related to their sexual identity in this unconscious, imitative way. Among traditional peoples, the tribe or social collective prescribed how men and women should interact. Since individuals did not have to question or even think about male/female roles in such cultures, the relations between the sexes were able to function smoothly and unconsciously.

In our culture, the predominant stereotype portrays a strong, protective male and a soft, compliant female. Whether we regard these roles with nostalgia or with horror, they no longer seem to be viable models. Cut off from masculine strength, women often become passive, dependent types who desperately try to attach themselves to men. Cut off from their feminine sensitivity, men become brittle and overbearing, lacking in vision and depth. And couples who try to live out conventional stereotypes of domestic bliss often wind up sadly disillusioned. Nonetheless, feeling the pain of these dead ends can provoke us to explore our masculinity or femininity in a deeper, more conscious way.

STAGE TWO: DEVELOPING A BALANCE OF MASCULINE AND FEMININE WITHIN

To be individual is, literally, to be "undivided, whole." So to find an authentic individual style of being male or female, we need access to the whole spectrum of masculine and feminine energies moving in us, beneath any stereotypes of manliness or womanliness.

This means exploring and cultivating certain qualities previously considered the province of the other sex. When a woman, for instance, decides to face life as an individual, rather than as a man's appendage, she naturally begins to develop qualities once considered masculine—such as autonomy, independence, or assertiveness. When a man feels stifled by the conventional codes of manliness, he naturally becomes more curious about his gentle, intuitive, receptive side. Although it may seem risky to try out these new qualities, the potential reward is a more balanced expression of masculine and feminine energies within us.

Cultivating this wider spectrum of energies also expands our vision. We begin to see how masculine and feminine are part of a larger interplay of polar forces at work in everything, down to the very spin of the subatomic particles. The ancient Chinese view of yin and yang is particularly useful in revealing how these two energies interact in all phenomena. By helping us see how there are two sides to *everything,* it can change our view of masculine and feminine from *oppositional* to *complementary.*

Yin is the energy of centripetal force, associated with inwardness, gathering together, cohesion, and relatedness. It is associated with the elements earth—the abundant ground that connects and sustains us as human beings—and water—the fluid, graceful mother of life. Like the generous, accommodating earth, yin nurtures the ripening of individual beings. Whether we are male or female, we can find sustenance in this power of connectedness. Its mature expression is earth wisdom or "old yin"—a seasoned knowledge that comes from working with things from the ground up. When we are in touch with this quality, we are not afraid to be ourselves. We can take our seat on this earth without apology or pretense, drawing on a power that comes to us from the depths. If we ignore this deep earth-body-wisdom and live mainly in our busy minds, we tend to shrivel up.

Yang is the principle of centrifugal force, separation, and individuation. Like a rocket exerting tremendous force to break away from earth's gravity, yang is the power that propels our development as individuals. It is associated with the expansive elements, air and fire. Yang is the energy of fertilizing, initiating, and executing. It is piercing, penetrating, and arousing, like thunder and lightning. And its mature expression is heaven wisdom: the ability to expand beyond narrow viewpoints and to see one's life in larger cosmic perspective. While yin governs coming together, yang governs moving apart. These two poles of human relationships are the basic principles governing all interactions in the universe.

Yin and yang are not confined to any single form of expression. We can see this in polytheistic religions, like those of ancient Greece or India, whose pantheons of gods and goddesses embody these energies in many different ways. For example, a scientist (Apollo) and a warrior (Mars) express yang in very different ways, just as a mother (Demeter) and a sensual lover (Venus) express yin differently. Polytheistic religions also portray yang qualities in women (Artemis, Athena) and yin qualities in men (Adonis, Pan). They recognize earthy male gods (Dionysus, Vulcan, the Celtic horned gods) as well as heavenly female goddesses (Ishtar, the Queen of Heaven, and the sky-dancer dakinis in the Tibetan tradition).

So we cannot strictly associate yin and earth with women or yang and heaven with men. In the area of emotional expressiveness, for instance, women are often more yang—initiating, provoking, penetrating—than men, who are often more passive, shy, or hidden with their feelings. As an ancient Chinese medical text states, "Both man and woman are products of two primary elements, hence both qualities are contained in each sex."

Nonetheless, men generally contain a larger proportion of yang, and are said to "belong to yang." Women generally contain a larger proportion of yin, and are said to "belong to yin." In other words, yang is "home base" for men, and yin is "home base" for women. Thus a man could be earthy and sensitive, but unless he is also in touch with yang energy—his fiery initiative or expansive vision—his masculinity will be incomplete. And a woman could be a strong leader or a brilliant thinker, but unless she is in touch with her earthy receptive qualities or her watery intuitive side, something will be missing from her femininity.

Thus it becomes clear that men and women cannot ripen fully into themselves unless they develop both yin and yang within them. A woman who is yielding and nurturing, but cannot act on her own or think for herself, is not yet fully developed. She may have "young yin"—and be girlish, attractive, and sweet.

Yet developing her yang side can help her tap a deeper kind of female power. When she can stand up as an individual, she can also sink deeper roots into her earth-wisdom, developing "old yin" sagacity and prowess.

Similarly, the classic macho male who has to prove that he is a "real man" is still unripe. As long as he fears opening to his softer yin side, he will never grow up. He has "young yang"—he can be bold and aggressive—but he has not yet ripened into "old yang," the real power and wisdom of manhood. Young yang is green and raw, very full of itself, like a new shoot pushing up through the earth. Yet if this shoot is to grow into a tree that can bear fruit, it must go through a yin stage of opening and receiving—light from the sun and nutrients from the earth.

Now that women are turning their energies outward, it is not surprising that many men have started turning inward, seeking new sources of guidance through meditation, psychotherapy, or just plain soul-searching. When a man becomes more receptive, rather than trying to control or manipulate, he develops a larger vision of life, which is the hallmark of old yang wisdom. A man becomes truly wise only when he has integrated his yin side.

Yet because oppositional mind runs so deep, we may find that in overthrowing the hold one side has over us, we become dominated by the other side instead. Thus, in cultivating gentleness and receptivity, and in reacting against old macho stereotypes, many modern men have turned against their male power altogether. As their newfound yin sensitivity takes them over, they are unable to take forceful stands or express strong convictions. Robert Bly has described such men as "soft males," who are lacking in energy, "life-preserving, but not exactly life-giving." There are times when a man must be able to bend and yield, but at other times he must be able to take charge. If a man's sensitivity undermines his yang strength, and he cannot express firmness or leadership, this only creates a new set of problems in his life and in his relationships.

A similar danger exists in reverse for many modern women. A woman's newfound yang power may attack or eclipse her feminine softness, making her brittle, hard, and inflexible. Taking on the brash quality of young yang, she adopts the same negative bias toward the feminine that has oppressed women throughout history, and so loses touch with her native feminine powers. This has a disruptive influence on her intimate relationships. And she misses the larger purpose of cultivating her yang power—which is to overcome one-sidedness and become a fuller, richer human being.

Another potential hazard in cultivating both yin and yang within ourselves would be to conclude that men and women are not really different. Couples who water down their differences, overemphasizing how they are both "just people" or "pals," create a unisex blandness that lacks passion and vigor. Androgyny—the complementary expression of masculine and feminine within each individual—can be an important stage. However, when used as a way to avoid the sharp edge where male and female differences rub up against each other, it can lead to a dry sort of companionship that lacks creative spark and sacred depth.

Finding a graceful balance between masculine and feminine ways of being is never easy. Just as a dancer has to work hard to develop spontaneity and grace, so learning to dance in a balanced way with the full spectrum of our sexual energies takes practice. We have been out of balance for so long that we can expect to fall into extremes along the way. In this light, the rigid man, the passive woman, the soft male, and the hard female *all* have further to go. They all manifest incomplete stages in a larger development.

In the end, a relationship can become richer, more spontaneous, and more adventurous when neither partner has a monopoly on either pole of tenderness or toughness, receptivity or power. Then not only can the masculine energies in the man dance with the feminine energies in the woman, but the feminine in the man can play with the masculine in the woman as well. A man might exert an earth influence on a woman through his steadiness or support, and help settle her down. And a woman might bring in a heaven influence, arousing and stimulating her man by providing a larger perspective in certain areas. When the young yin and yang are strong in a woman and a man, their energy as lovers will remain vital; no matter what their age, she can be the playful heroine/maiden, and he the gallant hero. Yet at other times she might express young yang—by being boisterous or pursuing him sexually—while he might express the softer sensitivities of young yin. Finally, the interaction of their old yin and old yang would allow them to be parents or wise friends who can offer each other counsel and support.

In opening to this wider range of interactions, the play of man and woman develops a much richer texture and counterpoint than just two-part harmony. Men and women today can no longer afford to yield their "other half" to each other.

STAGE THREE: DISCOVERING THE GENUINE, POWERFUL MALE AND FEMALE

Beyond social conventions of manliness and womanliness, and the universal principles of yin and yang, what does it mean to be a man or a woman in the deepest, truest sense? Our essential maleness or femaleness comes to us from beyond the realm of the personal and affects us in ways we can never entirely formulate or comprehend. As Alan Watts put it, "What a *real* man or woman is always remains inconceivable, since their reality lies in nature, not in the verbal world of concepts." The further we go in exploring this question, the more we touch on a profound unknown, the sacred mystery of the sexes.

Nowadays we often imagine that it is more of an honor to be seen as "a person" than as a man or a woman. Yet our "personhood"—a term derived from *persona,* meaning "mask"—is but the outer husk of who we are. It is our known self, a thought–image of who we are, which we present to others for their inspection and approval. Though our "person" may be respectable or impressive, as an outer shell it has no "juice." Nor does it allow us to connect deeply with another being.

Our deepest sense of being male or female comes from the

body, as our inheritance from the energies of earth and sky. As such, it is a direct link to the sacred order of the cosmos. Unfortunately, however, many of us have lost touch with the powers of nature that nourish this essential male or female deep within.

So to find our genuine, powerful male or female energies, we need to reconnect with the wild, elemental spirit that lives in us, underneath all our civilized facades. The human spirit, despite centuries of superficial domestication, retains a fundamentally wild quality. It is wild in the way that wind, rain, and sun are, *wild* in this sense meaning "untampered with; as it is, in itself." This elemental wildness is not something crude or primitive. It is, rather, a reality beyond personality or conditioning: the god or goddess living and moving deep within, whose power nourishes us like a clear, pristine underground spring.

Since we have few models in our society of the genuine, powerful male and female in action, and little guidance about how to bring these qualities into our relationships, we could look to mythology—the world's repository of timeless truths—for hints and suggestions. Yet we should not take these mythological images too literally, for our wild spirit can never be captured in any single representation. They are merely evocative pointers that can help us explore our own experience more deeply.

Mythological images of the "wild man" or "wild woman" suggest that the undomesticated spirit within us represents a deeper kind of consciousness, rather than a regression to something primitive. Wild gods and goddesses such as Dionysus, Ishtar, Shiva, or Kali are highly conscious beings. Their fierceness is a transformative force that cuts through superficial beliefs and artificial facades. Artistic renderings of these deities portray an intriguing quality: For all their fierceness, they appear to be completely at peace in themselves. They are not in the least hesitant or apologetic about who they are.

Tibetan (Tantric) Buddhism has a tradition of "crazy wisdom" whose guardian deities all display this quality of fierce repose. In this tradition, wildness is an advanced form of wisdom. Crazy wisdom literally means "wisdom gone wild." Yet one must first develop some wisdom before it can go wild, manifesting as natural, primordial simplicity and spontaneity. Likewise, we can tap our genuine, wild male or female power only after we cut through conventional images and develop the wisdom that grows out of a healthy balance of yin and yang energies. Thus the sublime face of the great Hindu god of creation and destruction, Shiva Maheshvara, is flanked by two other heads—one male and one female.

THE WILD SPIRIT OF MALE AND FEMALE

Deep male power is often symbolized by hair and, in many esoteric traditions, by the color white. Shiva's long hair is the legendary source of the Ganges River and its purifying power. Bound up in a topknot on the crown of his head, the wild man's hair signifies his connection with heaven wisdom, which he can attain only by leaving collective, conventional beliefs behind and setting out to find his own truth. A man's spiritual power lies in his ability to *transcend all phenomena*—to detach himself from purely personal concerns in order to explore a greater impersonal truth that lies beyond them.

The wild spirit in a man never lets him rest entirely content with what has already been accomplished. His longing for the infinite gives him a sense that there is always more to do, more to discover, "miles to go before I sleep." He is the pioneer and explorer who finds himself by continually moving beyond the borders of the known world.[1]

The wild male spirit also has a raw, earthy, sexual side, as portrayed in images of the Celtic horned gods. Horns represent a man's strength and phallic potency when he draws the power of earth up through his whole body. European woodcuts of the wild man with a coat of hair all over him also suggest that a man's power must be fully embodied. Unless a man works on joining the powers of heaven and earth in his daily life, he will not ripen fully into manhood. Seduced by high-tech gadgetry—new cars, the latest computers, bulldozers, guided missiles—or

else by mental abstractions, he will be unable to guide himself
or inspire others.

The dance of Shiva portrays the essence of male power,
which is both completely detached and completely engaged at
the same time. In one hand, he holds a drum, symbolizing the
music of creation; in the other, a flame, the power of destruction.
Shiva is "Lord of the Dance" because he can either create or
destroy, as the occasion demands, while also seeing beyond both,
to the greater totality from which they arise. He can dance and
make love with playful, passionate abandon precisely because he
has no investment in "the small stuff" of life. In case you wonder
how he does this, he smiles inscrutably and points with a third
hand to his upraised foot, signaling simply, "Let go."

When a man develops this power of detached engagement,
he can guide and direct, take a firm stand, and act on convictions
based on commitment to truth, without apology. He does not
become bogged down in materialistic concerns, but can play
with many possibilities. When he brings this power into a relationship, he can provide a strong, steadying influence that allows a woman to relax and blossom.

Wild female power is usually symbolized by blood and the
color red, which represent vitality and fertility. In the Hindu
tradition, the dark goddess-mother Kali, dancing with a necklace
of skulls, represents the great ocean of blood at the beginning
and end of life. The wild woman in the Tibetan Buddhist tradition—the wrathful/playful dakini, the "sky-dancer"—is often
portrayed drinking blood or dripping menstrual blood on a
mirror.

Blood symbolizes the circulation of energy, which maintains the vitality of our existence. It is also the cohesive element
binding all the different parts of the body together in a single
functioning whole. If earth is the common ground that connects
us, blood symbolizes the power of earth, which brings strength
and renewal. Drawing on this power, the wild female can be
fierce and "bloodthirsty" when necessary. She has no use for
bloodless activities, bloodless thought, bloodless relationships.
You will not find her installed in front of a television set or

speaking computerese. Nor does she tolerate dishonesty or self-deception. The dakini's unconditional passion consumes dullness and insensitivity in the heat of her fiery dance. If you are pretentious or hypocritical, she will cut off your head with her dagger and wear it in a garland around her neck. In contrast to male spiritual power, which has to do with transcending phenomena, the great spiritual power of woman involves *wearing all phenomena as ornaments*—celebrating the play of life's energies as intrinsically sacred.

We have little notion of this dynamic, awakening quality of wild female energy in our culture, especially in a form that is friendly to men. The images of female strength we are most familiar with—such as Artemis, the wicked witch, or the amazon—portray a stage of women's independence that is often hostile toward men. Images from other cultures present a different picture, however.

The red dakini is not a wild woman who, like Artemis, is aloof from men. Although she dances on a male corpse—suggesting that the wild female spirit has no use for the deadening side of a man's conceptual mind—she also holds the white staff of her consort—symbolizing her union with the masculine principle of skillful action. So, while trampling small-minded ego beneath her feet, she embraces genuine masculine wakefulness in her arms. Since the dakini embodies the vast, spacious quality of awareness that gives birth to awakened mind, she can be one of man's greatest helpers on the path of discovering his deeper nature.

Thus in directing her wrath at a man's insensitivity, his tendency to walk around half-asleep, or his inability to make real contact, a woman can have an arousing, awakening influence on him. "Wake up! Come alive! Be present here with me!" she screams, shaking him loose from the petty worldliness that prevents him from manifesting his real power. When a man first comes across this wrathful quality in a woman, she may seem quite ruthless to him. Yet the essence of such ruthlessness, beyond all the distorted forms it may take, is *wrathful compassion*. This is different from crude aggression, for it arises out of the urge to cut through obstacles to greater aliveness. It is anger with the heart open.

The genuine, powerful male or female who lives deep within is available to each of us. Unfortunately, most of us have learned to distract ourselves from the call of this wild wisdom. We are often afraid of looking beneath our familiar, comfortable persona and giving up our superficial, domesticated ways. Society also teaches us to fear this deeper part of ourselves. Western psychology has sometimes reinforced this fear by portraying the "depths of the unconscious" as a primordial swamp of animalistic impulses. For instance, the Jungian psychologist Esther Harding writes:

> Beneath the decent facade of consciousness with its disciplined moral order and its good intentions lurk the crude, instinctive forces of life, like monsters of the deep. . . . Were they left to function unchecked, life would lose its meaning, being reduced once more to mere birth and death, as in the teeming world of primordial swamps.

By contrast, it is the wild man in Thoreau who can proclaim:

> Dullness is but another name for tameness. As the wild duck is more swift and beautiful than the tame, so is the wild—the mallard—thought, which wings its way above the fens. It was because the children of the Empire were not suckled by the wolf that they were conquered and displaced by the children of the northern forests who were. . . . In wildness is the preservation of the World.

Men and women have a real need to feel the elemental, juicy quality of life in and through their relations with each other. Indeed, what we often first fall in love with is someone's free spirit, which appears as proud, solitary, and self-contained as a soaring hawk or a wolf roaming the plains. Yet though we find the wild hawk beautiful, we may also want to cage it, so that it will not fly away. Thus, consciously or unconsciously, we often try to domesticate our partners. Binding them to us and trying to make them fit our needs, we sever their connection to the roots of their power. A woman may give up her own separate friends, activities, and ways of being to please her man. Or a man may give up his solitude and come to depend on his woman for vital energy. In so doing, they lose the wild otherness and beauty that attracted them to each other in the first place. What remains are two domesticated *persons* who have lost the vitality and mystery essential to sustain a vibrant love.

The poet Rilke wrote that a healthy relationship is one in which two partners guard and protect each other's solitude. In a similar vein, a man and a woman can learn to guard and protect their own and each other's wildness. To do this, they must cultivate their own individual connection to the deepest powers of life, instead of primarily deriving their sense of aliveness from each other. Men and women who are in touch with their native powers can help each other honor their free, elemental spirit in their everyday relations. They can become powerful allies, helping each other awaken to these larger powers.

When a man's and a woman's wild energies meet, they are no longer just friends or lovers. They become *consorts*—which means that they have an energizing role to play in each other's development. A consort is someone who initiates us, through intimate contact, into certain mysteries we could not penetrate as readily on our own. In certain Tantric traditions, for instance, yogis would seek out a consort to help them attain a major aim of esoteric practice—joining the red feminine essence with the white masculine essence within oneself. The function of a consort is to help us awaken into the fullness of our being, using whatever means are necessary, whether through inspiring and enriching or through instructing and cajoling. This deeper kind of alliance is what men and women need to discover now.

Yet if we live mostly on the surface of our being, we cannot serve each other in this way. Instead, we will see each other's different ways of doing things as a problem. ("Why are you like *that?* Why aren't you more like me?") A woman's arousing nature will come across as bitchiness, while a man's ability to see beyond the personal will turn into a dry remoteness and emotional unavailability.

Women have great strength in the area of *personal truth* and *connectedness,* while men are strong in a different, complementary area—the ability to take and hold an *impersonal perspective.* A woman's thinking and feeling work closely together, giving her special aptitudes not only for intuition and empathy, but also for expressing what she feels, right on the spot. Men have a much harder time with this. Their strength lies more in detaching their awareness from their immediate feelings. (This difference may even have a physiological basis: the two halves of the brain, with their different functions, are more closely linked in women than in men.)[2]

Thus women often want more from their men in relationships—more intimacy, more closeness, more communication, more sharing of their inner life. The wild female spirit in a woman will continually provoke and inspire a man to be more direct, more honest, more vitally present, and more involved. This is her red essence at work.

Men need this, and can usually benefit from learning to relate in a more feeling way. Yet a man may find that a woman's way of acknowledging and expressing feelings is not always *his* way. If he is in touch with his elemental male spirit, he may feel a need to include a larger, nonpersonal kind of space in their relationship as well. He may even feel that too much closeness on a purely personal level diminishes the erotic charge between them. He may find that he connects with the wild woman in his partner more fully if they can also let go of relating as "persons" and interact in more elemental ways. This is an expression of his white essence, his Shiva nature.

When a man honors his wild spirit and brings it into a relationship, he can be more receptive to what a woman has to teach him about relating on a personal level. He can appreciate her ease in connecting as part of *her* native strength, a gift she brings to the relationship. Then she can help him—and he can welcome her help—in expressing and sharing his personal truth more freely. He can acknowledge that she is actually initiating him into a new area of his being.

He can also give her important gifts in turn. His desire to meet her beyond the personal level can help deepen their erotic connection and keep it fresh. He can help her free herself from getting bogged down in her emotions and lighten up when she becomes too serious. Because he is not so swayed by feelings, he can take charge of situations when she is at sea. When he comes from the ground of his creative male power, rather than from trying to control her or avoid his feelings, a woman can more readily follow his lead with confidence, and often with gratitude, for he is also initiating her into new areas.

When a man can celebrate his maleness, he feels more at home in himself in a relationship. Most women will find such a man completely attractive. The more she celebrates the essential female in herself, the more powerful and attractive she becomes as well. And this further inspires him to assume his power as a man. When the sexes honor their different qualities of spirit, instead of trying to convert each other to their own style as the "right way to be," their relationship develops greater power and depth.

As we move in this direction, we glimpse a new possibility—of men and women meeting in love and mutual respect, from positions of equal power, without having to either blame each other or apologize for who they are. At bottom, the deep, essential male or female in us *wants* to help our partner wake up to the full magnificence of his or her being. When the wild intelligence of man and woman mate with each other, the powers of heaven and earth also join, giving birth to more fully developed human beings.

13

Taming the Monsters

As we begin to move toward a deeper, more powerful man/ woman alliance in our relationships, many of us may come across a major obstacle: The wild male or female spirit in us may have been wounded or distorted in the course of our development. If a man's spirit has been crushed (perhaps by his father's abuse or his mother's invasiveness) or malnourished (by his father's neglect or failure to model strong male qualities), he will have a hard time finding and celebrating his genuine maleness or responding to the genuine femaleness in his partner. Or if a woman's father bullied her or bound her to him, instead of providing safety and protection, or her mother failed to model feminine strength, she may grow up distrusting both male and female power, and thus have a hard time feeling good being a woman in relation to men.

Such experiences create strong undercurrents of self-doubt and mutual distrust between the sexes. Often these appear in the guise of "monsters" that emerge unexpectedly, seemingly out of nowhere, at the point when a relationship is on the verge of moving to a new depth. Something furious inside us comes out fighting, savagely thrashing around, or else panicking and running away like a wounded animal. There are two main ways in which this wounded wildness seems to emerge, corresponding to the two poles of relationship: through aggression, which is a wounded way of making contact without having to yield control; and through isolation, which is a wounded way of creating space or separateness, by running away from intimacy altogether.

So if we are to deepen the male/female bond, it is not enough just to contact our wild spirit. We also must be able to "tame the monsters"—the distorted, negative forms our wildness takes—that so often tear relationships apart. When one person tames another, it creates a special bond between them. In Saint-Exupery's story, *The Little Prince,* the fox asks the Little Prince to tame him. He explains that taming means "to establish ties. . . . If you tame me, then we shall need each other. To me, you will be unique in all the world. To you, I shall be unique in all the world." Taming in this sense does not mean domesticating someone, fitting our partner into some narrow box. On the contrary, it is a way of softening the hard-hearted parts in each other, thus freeing our spirit so that it can contribute positively to the relationship. Men and women can do this by calling upon the warrior spirit within them and meeting these monsters with strength and resolve. Men need that from women, and women need that from men. This is part of their sacred alchemy.

TAMING AGGRESSION: THE GIANT AND THE WITCH

If a man cannot take a firm stand in his yang power with a woman, he may try to overpower and control her instead. This controlling quality is often personified in folk tales as the giant. The thickheaded, oafish male who is numb to his inner life throws his weight around without regard for others' feelings. If you happen to get in his way, he just tramples on you. Because he does not draw on his genuine strength, he cannot let himself be soft either. So he hardens himself by building a thick shield of armor that keeps him from feeling any tenderness. Many men in our society have some element of the oafish giant in them, which comes across as a gruff, callous streak. An extreme version is the rapist who seeks not intimacy, but supremacy.

If a woman does not trust the strength of her deep, feminine power, she too may try to protect herself through control and aggression. In folk mythology a common image of this hard-hearted tendency in a woman is the wicked witch, who usually eats people or casts spells to keep them in her power.[1] While the giant dominates through toughness and brutishness, the witch controls through cunning and trickery. The witch wants to harm men, unlike the dakini, who uses her fierceness to awaken them. This is because the witch is angry about being unable to be yin. She cannot trust the masculine to honor and protect that side of her.

It is important to understand that these elements are only fragments of our personality, old karmic residues, never the whole of who we are. For instance, when a man discovers a woman's hostile streak, he should not imagine that she *is* a witch. But if he wants her, he will have to tame that part of her, and thereby help free her young yin from the witch's spell. He may or may not be up to this task. If he is not, he may fall under the witch's influence and be subdued by her. To tame the hostile streak in a woman, a man must display genuine yang strength, courage, and willingness to stand his ground. If he is aggressive or domineering, he will only stir up the witch's wrath all the more. If he is passive or soft, she may eat him alive.

Kathy was a beautiful woman in her mid-thirties who had never found a man who was "good enough" for her. She seemed soft and warm on the surface, but when men got to know her, they found her strangely aloof and impenetrable. Her mother had been a successful businesswoman who had left her in the care of nurses. So from a very early age, Kathy suffered from lack of contact with a strong, nurturing feminine presence. As a result, she developed an identity built upon the story, "I can take care of myself. I don't need anyone."

Her father also had not been emotionally available. Out of his own insecurity, he was domineering, rather than protective or fatherly in the best sense. Yet Kathy idealized him, and her beauty won her the honor of being his favorite child. In her adolescent years, he would approach her a little too intimately, which scared and embarrassed her. So while her mother's distance left her distrustful of her own femininity, her father's unpredictable swings between being unavailable and overindulgent left her with a deep distrust of men as well.

Since Kathy did not trust male power, she would always try to test a man's strength at a certain point in a relationship. She would turn on him and hurt him in some deep way, sometimes by sleeping with someone else, sometimes by verbally assaulting him. Or she would often say the most outrageous things to see whether he could stand up to her. In this way, she was crying out for a kind of contact that could release her from her deepest fears. Would her partner buckle under when she screamed and shouted? Or could he handle her fury? This was the strength she needed to find in a man. Of course, neither she nor her lovers had a clue about what was really happening. She would even hate herself for becoming so aggressive, while her lovers would often leave in horror or defeat.

Eventually a man came along who could stand up to her. Somehow Paul was not daunted when Kathy's fierceness would emerge or when she would become cold and aloof. He saw these as distorted expressions of a wild beauty that he also loved in her.

Paul was able to tame her aggression by "holding the sword"—bringing his unflinching male strength to bear on the situation while also maintaining forceful contact with her. This did not mean *wielding* the sword—using his strength to bully, attack, or hurt her. When Kathy would start acting out her woundedness, Paul would hold his ground and let her know, "I'm going to meet this part of you head-on and not let you get destructive." Early in their relationship, when they would have a fight and she felt overwhelmed with rage, her way of hurting him was to walk out and not call or come back for days. As time went on, she would not stay away as long. Finally, one day when she was threatening to walk out and leave for good, Paul held her, sat her down, and told her, firmly yet lovingly, "You're not going anywhere. You belong right here. Take off your coat and stay awhile." After that, she never ran off again. Of course, this would not have worked if he were just imposing his will on her. But because he was showing her that he was really there for her, and that he was not afraid of meeting her with his strength, she could relent and soften.

By holding up his sword of discrimination—saying no to the negative witch and yes to the beautiful wild woman he loved—Paul was also helping Kathy distinguish between these parts of herself. By naming and standing up to the witch, he was protecting her—from her own fear and aggression. By meeting the genuine need behind her witchiness—to know that a man could really be there—he helped her come out and join him. And by showing her his yang strength, he helped her trust that she could be yin in relation to him. When she could count on him to be powerfully present, no matter how much she was lashing out, she could relax. She no longer had to fight against being a woman. This is how he tamed her.

A woman also can tame the aggressive streak in a man, but usually in a somewhat different way—through the power of gentleness. The angry feminist stance, which uses yang aggression as a weapon to attack male power, does not bring out the best in a man. When the yang in a woman attacks the yang in a man, it usually only makes him more aggressive. Or, if he does cave in, he may become "henpecked," which is the sign of a spirit that has been broken, rather than tamed in any positive sense.

It is important to distinguish true gentleness, which is grounded in strength, from passive compliance, which, because it is cut off from strength, may incite aggression instead of taming it. In the *I Ching*, the hexagram called "The Gentle" is also known as "the penetrating," thus indicating its dynamic, piercing quality.[2] This kind of gentleness, like water, can seep into and penetrate the cracks in a man's armor, awakening the deep, powerful masculinity within him.

Serge was a man whose aggressive streak would start to come out whenever he became deeply involved with a woman— he would treat her callously or insensitively in various ways. In childhood his father had not been around to protect him from an alcoholic mother, so he had developed this hardness as a defense, to keep his mother at a distance. He had already destroyed one marriage by relying too much on this defensive structure.

When Lynn first came into his life, she loved him very much, but couldn't figure out how to handle his aggression. She could see that underneath it he was afraid of being hurt, and that attacking him would only make him harden further. Her uncertainty about how to handle the situation brought her to the razor's edge, where she felt both the pain of his hardness toward her and her love for him. Drawing on the strength and presence that emerge when we simply open to our experience, however raw it is, Lynn was able to expose her pain *and* her love, without defense or fabrication. This enabled Serge to feel the quality of her love and see the effects of his callousness in a way he never had before. He admired her for the soft quality of strength she was expressing, and felt a desire to be worthy of her love. A sense of gallantry rose up inside him.

Through expressing a gentleness that was not just compliant, Lynn drew upon her deep feminine earth wisdom. Her strong, tender presence not only disarmed Serge, but also aroused an instinctive urge in him to protect her, from—what else?—himself. This forced him to look more deeply at his defensive patterns and see how he might behave differently.

Since aggression is hardness cut off from softness, to overcome it we need to bring these two qualities together in ourselves. Both Paul and Lynn, for example, used a balance of strength and gentleness to tame their partners' distortions. Yet there seems to be a general difference in the taming styles that work best for men and women. A man is usually more successful if his firmness is in the foreground, supported by an underlying quality of gentleness, while a woman is often more effective if her gentleness is in the foreground, rooted in an underlying quality of strength.

Of course there will always be times when the opposite style is called for. For instance, a woman may also need to hold the sword, stand her ground, and display her wrath, like the fiery dakini. Especially if a man is bullying or abusing her, she may need to protect herself by sharply confronting his aggression. Yet if a woman's general strategy is to attack a man's denseness through toughness and confrontation, she may cause him to back down, but she will never tame him.

Taming can happen only when we can get bigger than our partner's distortions. Therefore, if we are stuck in a lop-sided stage of our development as a man or woman, we will have a hard time subduing our partner's monsters. Neither the macho male who must prove himself nor the soft male who only wants to please can tame or outwit the wicked witch. A man can penetrate a woman's aggression only through expressing a balanced, mature strength. Similarly, neither the passive, compliant female nor the strident, aggressive one can penetrate a man's tough defenses. What gets through to him is a steady, gentle presence, which encourages him to let down his guard and expose his heart. The aggressive elements in us yield only when we see something larger in our partner coming to meet them—namely, the genuine, powerful man or woman.

In these feats of loving bravery, a man and a woman become allies who help each other ripen and blossom. Here we see the real, sacred alchemy of the sexes at work: When a man can powerfully express his maleness, he calls forth the authentic woman in his partner, and vice versa. This is the message we find in many of the world's folk tales. When a woman penetrates the heart of the giant in a man, when Beauty tames the Beast through her loving kindness, he turns out to be a worthy prince after all. When a man stands up to the domineering witch in a woman, he frees the princess from her spell, and she can then become his queen.[3] In facing these monsters lurking inside us with the courage of a warrior, we find that they are not as horrible as we had thought. As Rilke put it:

> Perhaps the dragons in our lives are princesses who are only waiting to see us act, just once, with beauty and courage. Perhaps everything terrible is, in its deepest essence, something that feels helpless and needs our love.

Our monsters are only masks worn by those parts of us that feel powerless or unlovable. They want, most of all, to be met and seen through.

WORKING WITH ISOLATION TENDENCIES

Since our aggressive tendencies are a wounded way of trying to make contact, these "monsters" can be transformed by someone making contact with us in a powerful new way. It is often much harder, however, for our partner to tame those parts of us that seek isolation or run from intimacy—the lone wolf, the Peter Pan, or the amazon.

The "lone wolf"—one who, in the words of a Robert Bly poem, "eats distance and silence"—cannot trust himself with women because he has not yet ripened as a man. Similarly, a woman who hardens into an amazonian "Who needs men?" stance usually has not fully ripened as a woman. Another way of isolating is by remaining a perpetual adolescent—what the Jungians call a *puer aeternus,* or eternal boy. This kind of male has brief and fleeting contact with women and may even be a Don Juan, flitting like a bee from flower to flower. The female counterpart is the *puella,* or eternal girl. The *puer* and *puella* have not developed the strength and confidence that would allow them to make real choices, root themselves on the earth, or be part of an ongoing committed relationship.

All these isolation tendencies are wounded ways of trying to create a space of our own where we do not feel overpowered by others. They indicate that we need to find or develop our own strength before we will be ready to contact others more fully. An intimate partner often cannot do much to remedy our incomplete development as a man or a woman. A man's love can help bring out a woman's feminine qualities, but only up to a point. Beyond that point, if she is not connected with her deeper feminine power, she may only be able to ripen and heal through contact with other women who can model and transmit the feminine qualities she is missing. Similarly, a wounded male may need to ripen and develop as a man through connecting with other men, who can model genuine yang power for him.

Unfortunately, men today often remain perpetual adolescents because they lack guidance from older, wiser males. Male power has been so abused and the wild male spirit has become so subjugated by the forces of materialism that we have difficulty finding older male wisdom we can respect. Our world is dominated by young yang run amok and fake male power, as seen in our fascination with weapons of destruction and our brash attempts to exploit the earth. We accord hero status to rock stars who make careers out of being rebellious kids, to macho cult figures like Rambo, or to men who spend most of their lives "off the ground," in corporate headquarters at the top of skyscrapers. What is "cool" today is to resist growing up, to be a "whiz kid" who thinks himself too smart and clever to join the ranks of adult men.[4] So it is not surprising that in most American households, a boy's father has little to transmit in the way of heaven wisdom or old yang power.

Without such a transmission, a man will fear female power or flee from it by denying that the earth has any hold on him at all. Seeking to rise above the earth, he becomes a "flying boy," like Icarus or Peter Pan. As a symbol, flying represents the folly and arrogance of young yang trying to imitate the heaven wisdom of old yang, without having to undergo the discipline of working with earthly constraints. The flying boy often comes from a family in which the mother turns to him for the juice she finds lacking in her husband. As a result of this attention, he always needs to feel "special." He may enjoy playing to women as an audience, but he is rarely capable of sustained intimacy. What a flying boy needs before he can come down to earth and engage with a woman is to connect with genuine male power.

In traditional cultures, initiation rituals conducted by a community of older males or by a spiritual teacher served to transmit old yang wisdom-power to younger males. Older men in tribal cultures would often take boys from their mothers as they entered puberty. The boys would live with them, dance with them, hear their stories—and go through difficult trials before the older males deemed them worthy of entering the world of men.

Although men today may have to engage in an extensive search to find an older male who can transmit authentic masculine wisdom, this is an important part of our development that we cannot skip over lightly. It also can help us connect more deeply with women. After spending a powerful week with a group of other men, one man I know remarked, "To my surprise, I found that relating with men helped me more than anything else in learning how to relate to women."

A man I knew with *puer* tendencies had a hard time after the arrival of his first son, when he could no longer have his wife's attention all to himself. Suddenly he was not the "special kid" anymore, but had to assume an adult role. What helped him through this crisis was his connection with his spiritual teacher, a man he deeply respected who had taught him that difficult situations are often the best opportunities for growth. By trying to put these teachings into practice, he managed to steady himself and gain perspective on his situation. Even though his teacher was not physically present, he was able to use this relationship to tame his tendency to bolt and run. This crisis proved to be a watershed in his personal development, and it also helped him give himself more fully to his marriage.

A woman may have to go through a similar journey before she can open fully to a man. Especially in a patriarchal society where women have been trained to please and serve men first and foremost, young women often flee commitment out of fear of being dominated and controlled. Or else they may turn against men altogether, hardening into a self-sufficient amazon stance. In order to go beyond *puella* or amazon tendencies, women may have to connect more deeply with old yin, with the dark feminine earth power. They may have to go through a period of not being nice and pretty, of discovering their rage, their grief, and their ability to stand on their own and face life as it is. They also may need to seek out a community of women with whom to share these experiences. Some have described this process as a "descent to the goddess," to the primordial roots of the feminine psyche, enabling a woman to develop confidence in her deep female nature. This in turn can enable her to come back and engage with men with a renewed sense of strength and self-acceptance.

OPENING NEW CHANNELS

As we free our wild spirit from the heavy load of karma or past conditioning that has distorted it, we open new channels through which our elemental male or female energies can flow more freely. As this happens, all the different areas of a relationship start to brighten up, becoming more lively and vivid. We make love with more intensity. We fight with more brilliance. We reveal ourselves more courageously. We feel moved to extend our love more fully into the world around us. And we lose interest in the war of the sexes, for we are too busy enjoying the dance.

14

The Awakening Power
of Sex

> The sexual act is not for the depositing of seed. It
> is for leaping off into the unknown, as from a cliff's
> edge, like Sappho into the sea.
>
> D. H. LAWRENCE

> The full splendor of sexual experience does not
> reveal itself without a new mode of attention to the
> world in general. As a means of initiation into the
> "one body" of the universe, it requires a
> contemplative approach.
>
> ALAN WATTS

COUPLES OFTEN ASK how they can keep sex alive and interesting after many years together. If we stop and think about it, this is a rather strange question. Who has ever heard a musician ask how to stay interested in music, or a poet complain about being bored by poetry? Because it involves the whole body, sex can offer a depth and intensity of feeling that matches or surpasses that of music or poetry. Yet we often imagine that we must continually find new lovers to maintain our passion. If a musician does not need to keep changing instruments to stay interested in music, why do we imagine that we need a succession of new bodies?

It is an ongoing challenge to remain conscious in an intimate relationship, to recognize and include the whole range of our feeling and perception. This is especially true in the sexual area. Since, as Lawrence suggests, sex is a leap into the unknown, it puts us on the razor's edge and leaves us without a mask to hide behind. This makes it tempting to develop a comfortable, automatic style of sexual behavior in order to avoid the sharpness of this edge and reduce anxiety.

Thus lovemaking often becomes a rote exercise, a fixed action pattern like the ritualized behaviors that animals perform. Intent on reaching the familiar destination of a "good" orgasm, we keep lovemaking confined to a narrow groove, creating tunnel vision. This causes us to lose our sensitivity to the whole range of subtleties and nuances that make each erotic encounter fresh and alive. Thus we fail to appreciate that sex too is a journey, and that we can linger and enjoy the scenery along the way. Lovemaking becomes predictable and stale; its springs in the depth of our being dry up. We become jaded, and feel we have to go looking for different partners to inject new life into the experience.

BRINGING NEW AWARENESS TO SEXUALITY

How then can we be more awake and alive in our lovemaking? How can sex serve as a channel for the wild male and female energies to keep entering and renewing our relationships?

To tap the sacred power of sex, we have to give up trying to make it a known quantity. Instead of trying to make it fit some convenient mold—as a form of recreation, or as a separate compartment of our lives, something that only happens in bed—we must assume an attitude of beginner's mind in the face of its mysteries. Then we can begin to sharpen our awareness of its subtler qualities, seeing how they permeate the *whole* of our interaction with our partner. As D. H. Lawrence put it:

> Sex, to me, means the whole of the relationship between man and woman. And the relation of man to woman is wide as all

life. It consists in infinite different flows between the two
beings, different, even apparently contrary. Chastity is part of
the flow between man and woman, as is physical passion. And
beyond these, an infinite range of subtle communication
which we know nothing about. . . . The relation of man to
woman is the flowing of two rivers side by side, sometimes
even mingling, then separating again, and travelling on. The
relationship is a lifelong change and a lifelong travelling. . . .
At periods, sex-desire itself departs completely. Yet the great
flow of the relationship goes on all the same, undying, and
this is the flow of living sex, the relation between man and
woman, that lasts a lifetime, and of which sex-desire is only
one vivid, most vivid manifestation.

Lawrence is speaking here of the subtle energetic flow between a man and a woman, which runs through all their interactions like a secret underground stream. Normally, we do not
notice this subtle level of exchange because our perception is
not that clearly or finely attuned. Instead, our mind is filled with
habitual expectations, beliefs, and response patterns. That is
why beginner's mind is important here—so that two people can
take a fresh look at how their energies interact throughout the
course of a day.

When we do this, we find that our style of emotional exchange has a strong effect on the quality of our lovemaking. If
our communication is blocked, if we are not honest with our
feelings, if we suppress or always act out our emotions, this
interferes with our subtle energy exchange and, along with it,
our potential for deep sexual communion. Thus emotional
honesty and clear communication are important steps on the
path toward greater sexual intimacy.

Beyond that, whatever we do to bring our wild spirit more
fully into our lives will deepen our sexual connection. For sex
loses its power when we domesticate it, making it serve personally defined ends, such as comfort and security. As Lawrence
suggests, the channels between man and woman must be "wide
as all life" if the most powerful energetic currents are to flow
freely through us. As long as we are just two "persons" making

love, the sacred power of sex will be diminished.

Unfortunately, our society teaches us to regard sexuality in a narrow, banal way—as a function of the gross physical body, rather than as a transformative energy that connects us with larger cosmic energies. For most of Western history, attitudes toward sex have swung between the extremes of repression/prudery and hedonism/debauchery—both of which promote a certain disdain for the body. From the prudish perspective, the sole legitimate function of sex is *procreation*, and the desires of the flesh are morally tainted. From the hedonistic perspective, sex is a form of *recreation*, and the body no more than a plaything. Since both these views fail to recognize the body as a sacred vessel, they prevent us from appreciating sex as a sacred activity. Thus sex and sacredness have been divided and set against one another for thousands of years in our culture.

Even the advent of modern sex theories has not helped the Western mind overcome its characteristic estrangement from the body. Freud's view of the purpose of sexual activity is still mostly banal: "to diminish the sexual tension and to quench temporarily the sexual desire (gratification analogous to satisfaction of hunger)." And his attitude toward the life of the body—which he regarded as a blind and brutish bundle of instincts, an "it" ("id") which threatens and undermines the "I" ("ego")—bears the typical Western stamp of alienation.

Although modern sex manuals finally brought the discussion of sexual practice out into the open, their emphasis on strategies, techniques, and prescribed goals also encourages the conditioned mind to maintain control over sexuality. They have promoted the image of an ideal "performance" of the "sex act," against which couples can measure themselves to see if they are "doing it right." Just in case you are unsure of how you measure up, you can now, in the words of a recent ad, even "consult a sophisticated computer program that analyzes your practices and fantasies in the context of the general population and puts all the most recent discoveries about sex *right into your computer.*" (D. H. Lawrence would have loved that!) The climax of the performance is, of course, orgasm, billed in the words of one popular sex manual as "the aim, the summit, the end of the sexual act." However, this tyranny of the orgasm makes sex an effort, creating what Masters and Johnson singled out as the most common cause of sexual dysfunction in modern times: performance pressure.[1]

The attempt to make sex into a procedure consisting of strategic techniques is like confusing musicology—the analysis of musical structure—with music itself. We can maintain a hearty enjoyment of sex, like music, only by immersing ourselves in the stream of its energy, letting go, and seeing where it takes us. If we want to keep lovemaking fresh, we need to put aside expectations and preconceptions, so we can be more sensitive to the changing energies and feelings arising in each moment of exchange with our partner. This is what will allow us to appreciate the unique, subtle shades and semitones in every erotic encounter. And, as the French novelist Balzac wrote, "If there are varieties (as of a melody) between one erotic occasion and another, a man can always enjoy happiness with one and the same woman." Thus, to stay interested in sex, we do not have to keep changing our sexual repertoire by collecting new partners or techniques. We need only our own open, wakeful presence.

SEX AND THE SUBTLE BODY

To sharpen our awareness of the subtle flows of sexual energy, both in lovemaking and in the everyday life of a relationship, we need to go beyond conventional Western views and appreciate this energy in a larger way. We can find such a larger view within the esoteric core of certain Eastern spiritual traditions, which see sexual energy not as a crude instinctual drive, but as the expression of a subtle life force animating the whole body. These traditions have even mapped the pathways in which this vital energy, known as *chi* in Chinese thought, or *prana* in the yogic traditions, flows throughout the body.[2] This energy flow and its pathways constitute what various traditions call the "subtle body," the "energy body," "the emotional body," or the "body of light."

In this view, vital energy can take many different forms, just as water can be either fluid, gaseous, or solid. The "solid," most readily perceptible form of vital energy is the gross physical body. Yet even the matter that makes up the gross body, as we know from modern physics, is not just solid, inert "stuff." It too is energy, always in dynamic movement and flux. Just as gross matter consists of finer pulsations of energy not observable to the five senses (physicists can only infer electrons, never see them), so the body contains finer, less tangible flows of energy circulating through it as well.

Yet though we cannot see people's subtle energies in the same way that we perceive their gross bodies,[3] we can, if we are sensitive, *feel* them—in colloquial terms, as the "vibrations" that people give off. Someone with a heavy, dark presence, for instance, conveys a very different feeling from someone who is nervous and excitable. Indeed, every person we know has a somewhat distinct "feeling tone" that interacts with our own subtle energy field in a unique way, generating attraction, interest, aversion, or indifference.[4] In the presence of some people, we feel a natural desire to open, while in the presence of others, we want to contract, pull back, or protect ourselves.

This sensitivity to the character of another person's energy field is an essential ingredient in sexual attraction. For instance, if a man is not attracted to a woman's energetic body (as measured by how he feels in her presence), any attraction he might have to her physical body will soon exhaust itself. Someone can be classically beautiful, yet not sexually magnetic if he or she is not energetically alive or present in the body. What is magnetic is not the body itself, but its vitality and vibrancy. In other words, the qualities of the subtle body—how we live in our physical body, the kinds of energy we express, how we touch and respond—are the key to sexual attraction.

How two people interact at this level—their "chemistry"— is the mysterious ingredient that can keep them interested in each other for a lifetime, in the face of difficulties that might

otherwise drive them apart. Without it, they may have everything else going for them, but they will lack the magnetism that
can hold them together. Regardless of how compatible two people might be physically or mentally, sex will soon lose interest
for them if they have no creative charge at the subtle body level.

When we make love, our subtle bodies interpenetrate in a
way that goes far beyond our exchange at the gross body level.
Only human beings make *love* through sex because only human
beings lie and linger front to front, with the softest parts of our
bodies fully exposed and in contact. At least two main feeling-
centers are located in the midsection of our soft front. The lower
center, around the navel, is the home of our "gut feelings"—
where we experience erotic resonance with another person. The
Chinese and Japanese consider this area (the *tan tien* or *hara*) to
be the body's center of gravity and seat of power. The upper
center is the area around the heart, where we sense more deli-
cate feelings of openness and surrender. Emotional exchange
also takes place through the eyes and mouth. While other pri-
mates copulate rapidly and from the rear, only human beings
exchange *chi*—the energy of their aliveness—by making love
face to face, belly to belly, heart to heart.

Thus two lovers' physical bodies are like musical instruments—they are the media through which the lovers' different
life energies weave a natural harmony and counterpoint. Just as
it is possible to pick up a musical instrument and make a random
assortment of noise instead of music, so two people can have
intercourse without it being musical or, in this case, intimate. If
there is no exchange of vital energy, they will be left feeling
empty, for they have used each other's bodies to create noise,
rather than song. Like music, sex can be used for utilitarian
purposes, for entertainment, or for meaningless background
filler. But it is most powerful when it awakens us to the rich, vital
textures and depths of human feeling. Sexual and musical expression both arise from the same place: from the energy flow
of the subtle body, which, by animating and shaping gross matter, is the source of creativity.

Since the subtle body cannot be literally pointed to, different traditions have developed symbolic ways of referring to its role in sexual magnetism. In some cultures, carrying a piece of a beloved's garment, to keep his or her scent present, is a way of maintaining attraction and fidelity. Scent is a molecular form of energy that can penetrate the apparently solid boundaries of gross matter, as when the aroma of perfume permeates clothing. Thus the beloved's scent reminds the lover of her subtle energetic essence, which he carries within him, even in her absence, all through the day.[5]

Other traditions speak of the blood-sympathy between lovers. When we say, "He's in my blood," or "I've got her under my skin," we are describing how our lover's subtle energy has mingled with ours. D. H. Lawrence describes sexual intimacy as a renewal of the blood, a "bringing together of the surcharged electric blood of the male with the polarized electric blood of the female, with the result of a tremendous flashing interchange, which alters . . . the very quality of *being,* in both. The blood is changed and renewed, refreshed, like the atmosphere after thunder." *Blood* in this sense is Lawrence's way of referring to the vital energy circulating through the subtle body. When he suggests that lovemaking alters and renews the blood, he is describing how it can penetrate our ordinary boundaries, open up blockages, and even out imbalances in our subtle energy flow.

SEXUAL COMMUNION: WOUND AND HEALING

As a form of subtle body communion, sexual intimacy cuts through the usual barriers and facades separating two people at the gross body level. The word *sex,* in fact, comes from the Latin word meaning "cut" *(secare, sectum).* And many cultures include ritual cutting—of the foreskin, the hymen, the face, an earlobe, hair—in initiation rites that mark the adolescent's entrance into manhood or womanhood. Sex cuts in the same way that meditation does: by shaking us loose from oppositional mind-sets and other mental distractions that keep us from feeling fully awake to the moment. When we experience it in this way—as a way of being present, rather than merely entertained—its sacred power can enter us. It strips away facades, exposing our pure, naked presence as nothing else can.

The cutting rituals that accompany many puberty rites also suggest something more: that we cannot enter the mysteries of sexuality unless we first acknowledge our wound—the basic ache of our separateness. Much as I might like to use lovemaking to help me forget my separateness, the sexual impulse arises out of feeling the contrast between myself and my consort, and gathers its potency from the play of our differences. Yet in allowing us to meet and connect beyond our conventional boundaries, sexuality also provides a healing. The erotic play of back and forth, in and out, soft and hard, shows us how to dance with our basic ache.

Similarly, when we sing or play music with someone, we join in a single stream of energy that lifts us out of our normal sense of separation, while the contrast between our different voices or instruments weaves a richer tapestry of sound than either of us could produce alone. So, in the act of love, a man and woman's subtle body fields join in a larger play of energy that lifts them out of their isolation and enriches them both, while also drawing on and illuminating the differences between their two natures.

The deepest moments of sexual communion are a sacred play of two-in-one, where all the polarities of life join together in a larger dance. Here in this sea of flux, the ebb and flow of opposites—rising and falling, tempest and harmony, surface and depth, friction and glissando, taking hold and letting go, fierceness and tenderness, power and vulnerability, heavenly inspiration and earthly pleasure—stream in and out of one another. When the polar energy fields of man and woman come together in this way, it is never just physical, emotional, or personal. Moments of deep sexual intimacy generate a powerful transfusion of energy from a level beyond our familiar ways of relating. As a man becomes pure male, a woman, pure female, the god and goddess enter.

Gods and goddesses in world mythology personify differ- ent primal energies at work in the natural world, as well as in our bodies. So, when the dark river god of the blood enters and moves in my body, I am no longer the familiar personality com- plex that I call "me." Instead, I am swept along on the stream of male power coursing through my veins, with its own rhythms and melodies, which I am hearing as if for the first time. My partner is no longer ego, but primordial woman, beyond time and space. In our lovemaking we could as well be lion and lioness, natives in the jungle, lord and lady, or dolphins in the sea. We are partners in the ageless dance.

In lifting us out of the narrow shell of personality, sexual communion puts us in touch with the larger energies of life flowing through our bodies. Thunder, lightning, electricity, rain, moonlight, and sunshine—the lovers who have not felt these energies in their lovemaking have not tasted the full rich- ness of sexual experience. In deep sexual communion, our worldly masks fall away and the living spirit can be felt and shared in its pure form.

Although this expansive awareness is not a substitute for spiritual realization—the full awakening to our unconditioned being, beyond the narrow confines of self—it can give us a powerful glimpse of that possibility. And it can inspire two peo- ple to bring a sacred quality of wakeful presence more fully into their everyday lives. This blood communion, which allows a man and a woman to discover themselves as god and goddess, is also the sacred basis for monogamy. As a pure expression of female energy, she is not just one woman, but all women; and when he becomes pure male, he can be all men to her.[6]

So when the modern mind reduces sex to a gross bodily function or to an animal instinct subordinated to the rational ego, it engages in a form of sacrilege. The more we try to define or manipulate sexual experience, the more we lose touch with its capacity to renew us and illuminate the heights and depths of human experience. We cannot fully appreciate its transformative quality unless we connect with our elemental wild spirit, which is forever unfathomable to the rational mind. In this mystery lies the awakening power and sacredness of sex.

15

Marriage as Mandala

MARRIAGE THROUGHOUT HISTORY has been primarily a worldly institution, designed to provide family cohesion and social stability and, more recently, personal happiness. Yet marriage no longer functions very well at delivering these "worldly goods." Given the fickleness of romantic feelings, the difficulty of getting along with another person, and the ease of divorce, it offers little guarantee of stability or happiness anymore. Nor does it confer any special status or cachet; for many people, even the words *husband* and *wife* have acquired a stodgy, boring ring. Thus marriage has become a major focal point of dissatisfaction. Some people complain that it no longer provides the security they seek, while others attack it as a faded relic from another era, an instrument of oppression, or a stifling arrangement that inhibits the natural appetites.

This situation brings up important questions: Why marry at all? Is marriage just an outdated artifact? Or does it serve some deeper human need and purpose? Apart from conventional social and religious beliefs, does marriage have a larger sacred function or meaning? Can marriage serve love's urge toward greater awareness, freedom, and truth, instead of being an instrument of torture, suppression, or deadening routine? What new source of inspiration can we find for marriage, beyond childrearing and hopes for perpetual romance or security?

THE CONTAINER OF MARRIAGE

Marriage is not just a pragmatic worldly arrangement. It also reflects a larger imperative of human life—which is to realize love's full potential by giving it an earthly form. Human nature is the intersection of inspiration and practicality, consciousness and matter, heavenly passion and earthly discipline. And marriage as a path provides continual opportunities to bring these two sides of life into fruitful union. Love without marriage is all inspiration, all passion. Marriage without love is all perspiration, all discipline. Neither of these situations allows us to realize the larger possibilities of the man/woman relationship. When a man and a woman blend the inspiration of love with the hard work of putting that inspiration into practice, their marriage becomes a sacred alchemy, joining heaven and earth.

Marriage involves the discipline of forging a container in which the love and passion between a man and a woman can ripen and bear fruit. Discipline always involves working with form. Form provides a vehicle through which we can put our passion and inspiration to work for creative purposes, so that we do not just squander these energies aimlessly. We may have great talent, but unless we cultivate a form of expression—such as writing, drawing, speaking, or playing a musical instrument—it will lack a creative outlet. Similarly, passion cannot be a creative path unless it is grounded in earthly form.

A couple I knew once wrote a book in which they argued that marriage involves a commitment to a *process,* rather than to any *form.* With this "process commitment," as they called it, if a couple is no longer growing, they should not feel obliged to stay together. Yet this approach is somewhat naive. If two people stay together only because their growth feels inspiring, then when that inspiration ebbs, going on together will become a problem. Commitment to growth without commitment to form is only a partial truth. The larger truth is that growth frequently brings two people up against extremely difficult issues that threaten to tear them apart as individuals and as a couple. Inspiration is essential, for it provides energy to work through these difficulties. Yet unless two people can also take on the practice of giving their love form, they are unlikely to go very far with each other.

This does not mean fitting a relationship into some preconceived mold. Rather, marriage gives love form by serving as an alchemical vessel in which two people's natures are steadily refined through the heat of their loving commitment to stand by each other: "We will not abandon or harm each other. We will not let our energetic connection leak or drain away, through carelessness or neglect. We will work out our conflicts within the container of our marriage, rather than letting them tear us apart. We intend to help each other develop our finest human qualities." This kind of intention and commitment helps us trust that it is all right to be completely open and exposed with our partner.

For this kind of trust to develop, we need a structure that can *contain* and *protect* the process of opening. If we turn to other lovers when things get hard, or complain to friends about problems in the relationship instead of confronting those problems with our partner, the container will be too leaky. And the potency of the connection cannot build. Marriage is a way of creating and sealing a container, so that the energies cooking within the relationship do not drain away.

By bringing all the different parts of ourselves into alignment with our highest intention, the marriage vow establishes the boundaries of this container. We all have parts of ourselves that do not want to bother with things that are difficult. Especially in our affluent society, we want to feel free to walk away from anything at any time. Yet because marriage is about the *realization* of love, not just its inspiration, it calls on us to deal with our fears of the earth—of becoming tied down, losing our freedom, having to deal with limitation and necessity. In taking a vow, we begin to subdue these fears and bring them under the yoke of our higher intelligence. We pledge that when things get hard, we will bring our combined energy to bear on the difficulties and see them through.

Of course, vowing to face whatever comes up in a marriage

does not mean that we will always execute this vow perfectly. How could we possibly do that? We cannot really discover what such a vow means until we have already been married for some time. We can learn about it only through practice, trying out new ways of being, making mistakes and giving ourselves tremendous room to learn. While the marriage vow cannot guarantee that we will always handle everything that comes up, it does signal our intention to make the attempt.

This kind of commitment is important because marriage is not just a connection between two people's beings, but also a juncture where, in the words of a Zen marriage ceremony, "two streams of karma become joined." When we marry someone, we also say, "I'm willing to take on your karma as part of what I am working with." Loving our partners "in sickness and in health" means not only accepting their larger being, but also staying open to them in the midst of all their karmic obstructions, even those that create pain and conflict.

Indeed, a marriage is unlikely to be transformative without a certain measure of pain and strife. Often only forceful confrontation can touch deeply ingrained patterns of fear and aggression, which rarely give up without a fight. When the heat of a couple's strife is contained by their commitment to marriage as a practice and a path, it can generate greater consciousness instead of blowing their relationship apart. A couple's willingness to work with each other "in sickness and in health" creates a sacred context for their conflicts, so that their fights can act on them, touch them, soften them, make them see new things about themselves they might not otherwise have seen, and thus deepen their connection.

When contained in this way, even our fights have a sacred quality, since they boil up out of the alchemical exchange that is happening between us. As the Tantric traditions suggest, when a man and a woman dedicate themselves to developing greater consciousness, then "the emotional vicissitudes of their personal relationship, the love and hate, the pride and jealousy, *are* the dakini's fine ornaments."[1] The dakini, as discussed earlier, represents the forceful quality of wakefulness that shakes us up and rouses us from our delusions. So when turbulence arises between two people who are using it as a tool to wake up, that chaos can be regarded as awakening mind in action.

Fortunately, the practice involved in working with form is not just hard work. It also helps us relax, give birth to new qualities of being, and realize new inner freedom. The more a musician practices his instrument, for instance, the more fully and freely his talent can express itself, without having to struggle with the limitations of technique. Through his practice and devotion, he masters not just technique, but, more importantly, *himself,* developing the inner confidence and sensitivity that will allow him to interpret his music in a masterful way. Similarly, the practice of meditation can help us realize the intrinsic wisdom and freedom of the mind—this, the very same mind that can drive us crazy when allowed to run on in an undisciplined way.

The practice of marriage works in the same way. Choosing to create a life and a path together helps my partner and I relax with each other; we no longer have to try so hard to win each other's approval, prove ourselves, or defend our separate territories. This frees up our energy to explore new areas, to cultivate deeper qualities of our being and see how to bring these more fully into our daily life.

MARRIAGE AS MANDALA

Whenever two halves of life come together—consciousness and form, passion and discipline, male and female, heaven and earth—a new world of possibilities comes into being. In this sense, two people joining their lives in marriage are engaging in a sacred activity because they are creating a cosmos in miniature—where all the different sides of themselves, personal and transpersonal, can be included. Before marriage, a couple's association is still loose and informal because it lacks clear boundaries. Taking a marriage vow creates a formal boundary, establishing the relationship as a sacred space where all the elements of life can interact and find expression.

The Eastern traditions use the term *mandala* to describe this kind of sacred microcosm. Mandalas have been portrayed visually in many different times and cultures as circles with four directions and a strong central focus. These symbols of totality and integration turn up in Paleolithic drawings, in Hindu and Buddhist sacred rituals, in sand paintings of the Pueblo Indians, as well as in medieval paintings of Christ surrounded by the four Evangelists. C. G. Jung also found mandala-like images spontaneously appearing in his patients' dreams as they were moving toward greater wholeness. A mandala portrays the conquest of oppositional mind, by bringing together life's polarities around a central unifying principle.

A mandala is a "cosmos" (literally, an "orderly world") because it is large enough to contain and handle chaos; thus it is "orderly chaos," in Chögyam Trungpa's words. When a man and a woman join their lives in marriage, they bring together a mix of many different, often contradictory influences; thus what comes up between them is bound to be chaotic. Marriage as a mandala is a formal practice of containing this chaos, so that it can enlarge, rather than destroy, their relationship. The chaos of relationship can become workable when a couple creates a sacred context around it, by setting boundaries and agreeing on a central governing principle—such as opening the heart or waking up to their deeper potential—to guide their life together.

In this way, the practice of marriage is akin to meditation. As you sit still and become more present to your experience, all the chaos of the mind arises. A flood of thoughts, feelings, fantasies passes through you. Your whole life passes before your eyes. It's total chaos. Yet the form of sitting practice—maintaining an upright posture and following the breath—creates a boundary that allows this chaos to be contained. And returning to the still, sane presence of awareness provides a central focus, which differentiates this practice from just letting the mind go wild. Because your mental chaos is contained in a formal setting, you can bring your attention and consciousness to bear on it, see through it, and learn to tame it. Without such a form, you are simply subject to the vagaries and wanderings of the mind.

Similarly, marriage, as a sacred microcosm, both invites all our chaos to come up and enables us to work with it more consciously. This allows a man and a woman to draw on all the turbulent energies arising out of their interaction as fuel for their journey. So instead of trying to make marriage fit some conventional image of harmony, we could welcome its power to expand our world. Regarding marriage as a mandala helps us take heart: If all kinds of wild energies and karmic eruptions arise in this space, that is not a problem. It is all part of the dance.

SACRED ORDER

So far we have seen that the formal commitment to marriage creates a boundary and a container that helps two people work and play with the energies arising between them. Yet something more is needed to create a mandala—a central governing principle. What is the central principle in the marriage mandala that can help make the chaos contained within it workable? In the Tibetan Buddhist tradition, the focal point of a mandala is always enlightened wisdom, symbolized by a deity at the center, surrounded by all the elements of the universe. This suggests that if two people are to make good use of the chaos arising between them, and not become overwhelmed by it, they must accord wisdom and truth a central place in their relationship. Then the natural order of things can unfold, for a sacred order has been established.

The original term for sacred order is *hierarchy* (from the Greek *hieros*, sacred, and *arche*, order). When most of us hear the term *hierarchy*, we think of a vertical pecking order, with a big boss at the top. Such a structure represents a debased form of hierarchy, however, because wisdom is not the organizing principle. For instance, in the patriarchal family, the wife and children had to submit to the decisions of the father or grandfather who was in charge, whether he was wise or foolish, right or wrong. For obvious reasons, that kind of "domination hierarchy" has been tremendously destructive and no longer works.

To establish sacred order in today's egalitarian marriages, we need a more flexible kind of arrangement, one that encourages both partners to realize their larger potential. For this, we could draw on the pattern found in all life forms—where more evolved structures (such as bodily organs) govern and integrate the functions of simpler structures (such as cells), thus promoting a higher level of overall functioning. This kind of "actualization hierarchy"[2] is what we find in a mandala, which, like a cell, contains a strong center around which peripheral elements organize themselves. How might this kind of life-affirming hierarchy work in a marriage?

First, a couple would recognize some form of wisdom or wakefulness as a central principle governing their union. Second, they would acknowledge that neither of them has exclusive access to this larger sanity; instead, each of them has different areas where they are strong or weak, clear or confused, insightful or blind. Third, recognizing and respecting each other's natural strengths, they would be willing to let the partner who has greater wisdom or clarity in a given area take the lead. For instance, if a woman has greater emotional flexibility than her man, then he would recognize her as his teacher in this area. He would let himself learn from her wisdom, instead of trying to force her to go along with his emotional rigidity. This is what it means to recognize her as his *consort*, someone who is in his life to help him grow. In this way, by recognizing, respecting, and learning from each other's natural strengths, two partners establish sacred order in their marriage.

When a man and a woman do not honor and respect each other's innate wisdom and strength, they disrupt natural hierarchy in their relations. For instance, a man who does not express appreciation for his wife's feminine qualities, who scorns the ways she is not like a man, who uses his yang power to dominate and criticize her, undermines the woman in her, thus destroying any possibility of a creative alliance between them. Or if a woman tries to cut down her husband's male power, she is undermining his yang and diminishing the real juice in their connection. When natural hierarchy is destroyed, the resulting disharmony will adversely affect every member of the family.

SURRENDER

Honoring each other's wisdom and strength means that both partners must be willing to surrender when the occasion calls for it. Indeed, marriage teaches us a great deal about the importance of surrender in our life as a whole.

The notion of surrender is widely misunderstood in our culture, and, like commitment and intimacy, often brings up fear. It conjures up images of "come out with your hands up"— waving a white flag, admitting defeat, losing power. Yet, if we understand it rightly, surrender does not have to mean giving up power or freedom. As an act of putting wisdom and truth above our personal ambitions or beliefs, it helps us align ourselves with the natural order of things.

The ability to surrender is central to any graceful or creative activity. Whether we are appreciating the sights, sounds, and tastes of the world, dancing, making love, or simply listening to another person, life continually calls on us to yield control and to open to what is beyond us. We cannot ultimately control what happens to us or have our way on this earth, if only because we must eventually give up everything and return to the great unknown from which we spring. Surrender involves letting go— of what we already know or have—and letting be—opening to the situations that life presents.

Many people distrust the notion of surrender because they confuse it with *submission* to another's will—which can in fact have disastrous consequences in a relationship. Submission means giving over power to someone else, putting that person above us while putting ourselves down. People often do this when they feel unworthy and in need of validation. An employee submits to his boss in order to gain recognition, favor, or a promotion. In a relationship, one partner might sacrifice his or her true direction or path in life to win approval, acceptance, or simply peace and quiet.

Of course, marriage does require real sacrifices. We cannot be as free and independent as we were before, and we are continually called upon to give, often at the most inconvenient times. Yet we should distinguish between two very different kinds of sacrifice. When we knowingly choose to give up something for a greater good, this is *conscious sacrifice,* which helps us grow and thus empowers us. However, when we try to please or placate by blindly going along with someone or bending ourselves out of shape, this is *neurotic sacrifice*—a form of submission that only debilitates.

In marriage, we can distinguish one from the other in the following way: Submission involves distorting who we are in order to win something in return. When we submit to someone, we give away our power and hope for the best. Surrender, on the other hand, requires discriminating awareness—recognizing a larger truth or following a direction that leads toward greater aliveness—rather than blind hope. When we surrender to what life situations call for, real power, which comes from beyond our personality, can enter us. While submission occurs out of inner weakness, genuine surrender can happen only out of feeling strong enough to take a risk.

The essential surrender in marriage is not *to our partner* as a finite personality. Instead, it involves opening ourselves to what the relationship has to teach us from day to day. As a marriage grows and develops, it provides continual opportunities to practice surrendering: by yielding to our partners' wisdom and opening ourselves to learning from them in areas where they are more wise or healthy; by giving ourselves more fully to the relationship; or by letting go of fixed attitudes and positions that prevent love from flowing freely. We can usually tell that some kind of surrender is called for when our standard operating procedure is not working, and our partner or the situation itself is calling on us to give it up. This might involve something as simple as recognizing that we have acted in a hurtful or stubborn way and saying, "I'm sorry." Such moments provide rare and powerful opportunities to break out of old karmic patterns.

The following examples illustrate three different kinds of surrender.

Eric felt awkward in social situations, while his wife, Robin, was more socially adept. At first, Eric tried to make his shyness the guideline for their relations with the outside world. As a result, they spent very little time as a couple with other people. By forcing Robin to submit to his fears in an area where she was more evolved than he was, Eric upset the natural hierarchy in their relationship, eventually creating a breach between them. After many fights, Eric finally saw that he needed to surrender control and let her be his teacher in this area. Although yielding to her guidance brought up anxiety and uncertainty, it also forced him to extend himself in new ways. This broadened him and enriched their relationship.

After twenty years of marriage, when a new depth of feeling opened up between Laura and her husband following a tragic family incident, she began to see that she had never given herself fully to their relationship. Yet she was unsure whether she could take the risk involved in becoming more open to him. In her words:

> I feel scared now that we have a new opportunity to be more open and loving together. I sense an immensity there that I almost don't want to see or touch. It feels so immense that I could get carried away or lose myself in it. Talking about it makes it sound wonderful, but the actual feeling isn't. . . . It's like a joy I almost don't want to permit myself. If I had that kind of joy, I'd be afraid it could get taken away. If I open to Daniel, how could I rely on him to be there? What if he died? How could I bear to let myself be that vulnerable?

These are the questions of someone on the razor's edge, feeling both the fear and the excitement of opening to unknown possibilities. Laura had no guarantee that opening up more with her husband would be safe. Yet she made the choice to move in this direction because it led toward greater aliveness.

Late one night Alex and his wife reached an impasse in a fight they were having. She just wanted to go to bed, while he was desperately worrying, "How can we work this out? If we love each other, why can't we solve this disagreement? If we can't resolve this, something must be wrong with our relationship. She should stick with this and not just go to bed." Yet the more he pressed for a resolution, the worse everything felt. In his words:

> I didn't know what to do. So I just let the situation be, and waited to see what would come of it, instead of trying to push through it—which was my usual style. This put me in a place where nothing made sense, where my ideas about how things should be were blown: "I thought Donna was like this, and she's not. I thought our relationship was like that, and it's not. I thought I could resolve anything between us, and I can't." This was one of those rare times when I had to admit that I couldn't understand, that life is bigger than what I could make out of it. Something snapped inside me. There was a moment of just letting go. Later it was followed by a sense of gratitude: "Our relationship is big enough to handle this. I'm so glad that I don't have to try to make everything right." I had discovered a new kind of trust. We went to bed, and the next day things felt much better between us.

Surrendering for Alex in this situation meant not trying to push ahead with his customary way of resolving differences, no matter how well it had worked before. Since the situation did not fit his usual logic, it was calling on him to back off and just let things be.

Surrendering does not mean always going along with whatever is happening. Nor does it mean that if a situation makes us angry, we should say to ourselves, "I shouldn't be angry, I should surrender." That would be suppressing ourselves, which could be a form of submission. If our usual pattern is to suppress our feelings, then maybe we need to surrender to our experience of anger. However, if our habitual style is to vent anger or use it to control others, then surrendering might mean putting aside our anger and approaching the situation in a more gentle way.

In each of these examples, one partner's act of surrendering opened up a stuck point in their relationship. Eric, Laura, and Alex were each being called on to let go of their standard operating procedures—which was frightening because it brought them to the edge of the unknown. Yet their willingness to open at those moments invited a certain natural wisdom into the situation, revealing new directions just when things seemed most scary. New order was born from seeming chaos.

DIMENSIONS OF MARRIAGE

Appreciating marriage as a mandala helps us understand that it is more than just a worldly arrangement. The Buddhist tradition recognizes mandalas as having three dimensions—outer, inner, and secret. The outer aspect of a mandala is how it manifests— its structure and form. The inner aspect of a mandala is what goes on within it—its meaning and energetic qualities. And the secret aspect of a mandala is how it affects and acts on us in subtle, less visible ways. Similarly, marriage is not just unidimensional, but works on several different levels at once.

The outer dimension of marriage is its socially recognized form: man and woman joining together in a lifelong partnership. This form is sacred because it belongs to the whole human community and is part of the human search to create a wholesome way of life. Wendell Berry describes the outer marriage when he says, "Forms join generations together, the young and the old, the living and the dead. Thus, for a couple, marriage is an entrance into a timeless community."

The outer mandala also includes creating a home or living space that expresses the character of a couple's connection. When two people attend to the details of their environment, their home enriches both themselves and everyone else who enters it. However, if they neglect their environment and leave it in disarray, this will magnify the disorder in their relationship as well. How life proceeds in the home, how a couple set up the schedule of daily life, reflects and affects how they are with each other. Do they get up and run off to work, come home, throw some food together, turn on the TV, and jump in bed? Or does their way of life express more elegance and dignity? These are all important aspects of the outer dimension of marriage.

Traditionally, marriage has been defined solely in terms of these outer elements—as a social contract, as participation in a community, as the making of a home and family. Yet though the outer marriage is important and sacred in its own right, it is no longer enough by itself to bind two people together. What is more crucial today is the inner marriage—the nature and quality of a couple's connection and interaction. How do they regard and treat each other? How do they communicate with each other? How do they respect each other and honor their connection?

The inner marriage is like a garden; even though the outer circumstances, such as soil and weather, may be favorable, it must still be tended if it is to bear fruit. Unless two people tend to the quality of their relationship, it is likely to deteriorate from unintentional neglect. They become sloppy, little things slip by, and before they know it, they have built up tremendous antagonism and resentment. The garden has become choked with weeds.

Mutual respect is an essential ingredient of the inner mandala. Respect involves recognizing that a human being has a great spirit, which reaches far beyond the familiar facade of personality we may know or see. If my partner and I always treat each other in a casual, familiar manner, relating to each other primarily as known quantities, we block the larger mysteries from entering our relationship. This causes us to lose respect for one another. Since marriage taps into larger energies beyond personality, this relationship can never be merely casual.

Because we are representatives in marriage of the elemental male and female, we could even regard each other as king and queen. A king and a queen treat each other with great dignity and respect. That is part of their discipline. A little formality of this kind can wake us up from the cozy familiarity that tends to envelop a long-term relationship. For instance, since men and women wear very different clothes when dressing up, occasionally dressing more formally can be a way to express and emphasize the different principles we represent. Dressing up is like polishing our qualities, so that they shine forth brilliantly, unobscured by the dust of everyday casualness. Many of us in present generations have rebelled against any kind of formality, perhaps because our parents or elders were formal in a stiff or sterile way. Yet marriage is a formal rather than a casual relationship. So a certain amount of formality, as a display of elegance and respect, can fan the sacred fire of a couple's love and brighten up the inner mandala of their marriage.

Finally, the "secret" dimension of marriage is the inner transformation that occurs as a direct result of two people's interaction. Within each individual a marriage is going on between yin and yang, heaven and earth, power and gentleness, and countless other polarities. This inner alchemy often precisely mirrors what is happening in the external relationship. For instance, caring for my partner forces me to see that I must also care for myself; commitment to the growth of the marriage also requires a commitment to my own growth; joining my life with a woman I love forces me to bring my own inner masculine and feminine into balance. The secret marriage involves giving up our old ideas about who we are, so that the different elements inside us can come together in new ways and we can keep being born anew.

All three of these dimensions of marriage—outer, inner, and secret—mutually enhance one another. If any of them are missing, a couple's life together will be that much poorer. Some couples may have a strong inner connection, but be unable to create a healthy, vibrant environment or lifestyle on the outer plane. Other couples may make a beautiful home together, while their exchange with each other remains shallow. When a couple can create a world together, relate to each other with passion and respect, and continually refine their natures through their interaction, their life together will be fertile and creative.

MARRIAGE AS REALIZATION

The easy part of any creative work is feeling inspired. The hard part is putting our inspiration into practice, embodying it in earthly form, for this brings us up against the limitations of the materials we are working with. A writer may have a grand vision of a book he wants to write, but finding the right words and format is always exacting and difficult. A pianist may know how he would like to sound, but getting his fingers to match his inspiration takes ongoing practice. Dealing with practical necessities and limitations is humbling. Yet it also gives birth to a richer kind of inspiration—which grows out of bringing vision into form.

The creative work of marriage is no different. It is easy to fall in love, but not so easy to put that love into practice. We keep coming up against the limitations of the raw materials—in this case, ourselves! The marriage commitment brings up levels of fear that we have never faced before. Yet in resolutely bringing our love to bear on the fears that threaten to constrict our hearts, we mine fresh sources of inspiration, much deeper than the first spontaneous sparks of falling in love. It is inspiring to see a man and a woman dancing with the energies contained in their chaos and helping each other open more fully to life. Just as an artist can affect others only through wrestling with his materials, similarly, a couple who can wrestle with the chaos arising between them develop a strength and humor that is heartening to others. Marriage, like a finished poem, is inspiration made manifest.

Many discussions of the difficulties of marriage today never go beyond the superficial and the mundane. They often focus on how hard it is for the modern couple to "have it all"— intimacy, commitment, children, two careers, child care, money, a home, and time enough to enjoy these things. Although these may be important practical concerns, merely finding a way to "have it all" will not save or renew marriage in these precarious times.

We can revitalize marriage only by re-visioning it as a sacred path. The sacredness of marriage is not handed down by family, society, or church. It arises out of two individuals' passionate devotion to bringing love into form. This involves taking each other on, no holds barred, in the spirit of "I accept you and am willing to bring my intelligence and heart to bear on all your rough edges; and I want you to do the same for me. Let us work on these things, and help each other realize the full range of our powers and possibilities." When a man and a woman join forces like this, all their ups and downs, their struggles and their joys, are held within a sacred context. Their marriage enables them to realize how "the two become one," how, despite all their differences and separateness, self and other, male and female, are of one spirit.

This vision of marriage as joining the two halves of life— the inspiration of heaven and the practicality of earth—has never been widely realized. The old model of marriage as a family duty was too earthbound, while modern attempts to "have it all" and "live happily ever after" are too naive and ungrounded. Perhaps only a small percentage of couples will be able to live marriage as an alchemical relationship that helps them give birth to their finest qualities. Nonetheless, both history and evolution have shown many times that even a few pioneers can forge a new direction, which points the way for countless others.

16

Conscious Love

> There is no necessary relation between love and
> children; but there is a necessary relation between
> love and creation. The aim of conscious love is to
> bring about rebirth.
>
> A. R. ORAGE

PEOPLE GENERALLY CONSIDER an intimate relationship successful
if it provides basic fulfillment in such areas as companionship,
security, sex, and self-esteem. Describing such an arrangement,
one of the characters in Woody Allen's film *Manhattan* provided
what *Time* magazine called a "reasonable definition of modern
love": "We have laughs together. I care about you. Your concerns are my concerns. We have great sex." Yet in regarding
relationship as path, especially as a sacred path, we hold a larger
vision, one that includes these needs, but is not limited to them.
Our central concern is with cultivating a conscious love, which
can inspire the development of greater awareness and the evolution of two people's beings.

Yet we should not be too idealistic about this, for intimate
relationships never function entirely on a conscious level. We
live on many levels simultaneously, all with different needs. The
tender child, the adventurous youth, the seasoned adult, and the
spiritual seeker are all simultaneously present in us. Intimate
relationships reflect this multilevel quality of our existence and
therefore never involve just one single kind of relatedness. To

clarify the part that conscious love can play in a relationship, it helps to consider it in the context of the many different levels of connection that can exist between two people.

LEVELS OF CONNECTION

The most primitive bond that may form between intimate partners is the urge for symbiotic *fusion,* born out of a desire to obtain emotional nurturance that was lacking in childhood. Of course, it is common for many couples, when they first get together, to go through a temporary symbiotic phase, when they cut out other activities or friends and spend most of their free time together. This stage in a relationship may help two people establish close emotional bonding. Yet if symbiosis becomes the primary dynamic in a relationship or goes on for too long, it will become increasingly confining. It sets up a parent–child dynamic that limits two people's range of expression and interaction, undermining the male–female charge between them and creating addictive patterns.

Beyond the primitive need for symbiotic fusion, the most basic desire in an intimate relationship is for *companionship.* This can take more or less sophisticated forms. On a crude level, we might just want another body around, almost like a pet, to share our bed or keep us company. On a more sophisticated level, the child in us wants a playmate, someone we can laugh and romp with, and the adult in us enjoys sharing activities such as cooking or attending cultural events together. Basic companionship plays a part in all relationships, although some people do not seem to want anything more than this from an intimate partner.

A further level of connectedness can happen when two people share not only activities and each other's company, but also common interests, goals, or values. We could call this level, where a couple begins to create a shared world, *community.* Like companionship, community is a concrete, earthy form of relatedness.

Beyond sharing values and interests lies *communication.* On this level, we share what is going on inside us—our thoughts, visions, experiences, and feelings. Establishing good communication is much more arduous than simply creating companionship and community. It requires that a couple be honest and courageous enough to expose what is going on inside them, and be willing to work on the inevitable obstacles in the way of sharing their different truths with each other. Good communication is probably the most important ingredient in the everyday health of a relationship.

A further extension of communication is *communion.* Beyond just sharing thoughts and feelings, this is a deep recognition of another person's being. This often takes place in silence—perhaps while looking into our partner's eyes, making love, walking in the woods, or listening to music together. Suddenly we feel touched and seen, not as a personality, but in the depth of our being. We are fully ourselves and fully in touch with our partner at the same time. This kind of connection is so rare and striking that it is usually unmistakable when it comes along. While two people can work on communication, communion is more spontaneous, beyond the will. Communication and communion are deeper, more subtle forms of intimacy than companionship and community, taking place at the level of mind and heart.

The deeper intimacy of communion may stir up a longing to overcome our separateness altogether, a longing for total *union* with someone we love. Yet though this longing expresses a genuine human need, it is more appropriately directed to the divine, the absolute, the infinite. When attached to an intimate relationship, it often creates problems. Putting our whole longing for spiritual realization onto a finite relationship can lead to idealization, inflation, addiction, and death (as discussed earlier in Chapter 6). The most appropriate way to address our longing for union is through a genuine spiritual practice, such as meditation, that teaches us how to go beyond oppositional mind altogether, in every area of our life. By pointing us in this direction, intimate relationship may inspire this kind of practice, but it can never be a complete substitute for it.

Every relationship will have different areas of strength along this continuum of connectedness. Some couples may share companionship and common interests, but have little real communication or communion; and some may have occasional moments of communion, but still find their strongest link at more basic levels. Others may share a deep soul-communion, yet have little in common on the earthly plane of community and companionship. Such couples might have a hard time creating a life together because they would lack simpler forms of related-ness to fall back on when the intensity of their communion wanes. Couples who share a deep being-connection, good communication, common interests and values, and a simple enjoyment of each other's company will have an ideal balance of heaven and earth connectedness. (Sexuality can operate at any of these levels—as a form of symbiotic fusion, as a body-companionship, as a shared sport, as a form of communication, or as a deeper communion.)

CONSCIOUS LOVE AND BROKEN HEART

Conscious love begins to develop in a relationship where two people share a being-to-being communion. This is because it is love of being rather than love of personality. In moments of communion, I am in touch with the depth of my own being and my partner's being at the same time. From day to day our inner lives also begin to move in synchrony. Her face becomes more familiar to me than my own. I become as sensitive to her changing moods and feelings as to my own. I share her longings and cannot separate myself from her pain. We have interpenetrated too deeply for me ever to be able to stand entirely separate from her again.

And yet, I *am* separate. No matter how close she and I are, we can never fully share our different worlds: She can never really know what it is like to be me and I can never really know what it is like to be her. Although we may share fleeting moments of oneness when our beings touch, complete union remains forever just out of reach. The closer we are, the more even a hair's breadth of distance between us seems like a huge ravine.

Nor is there any way to hold on to each other or use our closeness to shield ourselves from the truth of our aloneness. We are on temporary loan to each other from the universe, and we never know when it will claim us back. Feeling this edge—where we are neither entirely separate, nor entirely one—puts me back in touch with the rawness of the heart. In realizing that I can never completely overcome my aloneness by melting into the one I love, I am left with a basic ache from which no one can ever save me. Part of me would like to save her from her pain and make everything right for her, yet there is nothing I can do to shield her from her life or from our death. Here, where the heart feels both full and empty, I find the answer to the question posed by the modern love song, "Why does love got to be so sad?"

Yet this kind of sadness is not a problem. In Chögyam Trungpa's words, it "is unconditioned. It occurs because your heart is completely exposed." Love songs are so often sad in tone because devotion to another stirs a deep longing to melt and give ourselves away. As Trungpa puts it, "You would like to spill your heart's blood, give your heart to others." The word *sad* is related etymologically to *satisfied* or *sated,* meaning "full." Love's sadness is the *fullness of feeling* that arises out of our longing to open and connect. Thus at the core of devotion to another is a sweet, sad fullness of heart, which longs to overflow.

Since my aloneness is also what makes me want to overflow, it need not isolate me. As a simple presence to life, it is what I share with all the creatures of the earth. It is an inner depth from which many treasures arise: a passion to reach out, extend myself, write a poem or a song, give something of substance or beauty that could touch the one I love in *her* magnificent aloneness. Out of it comes the greatest gift I can give: myself, the whole of who I am, in all my desire to live and die as fully as I can.

Thus when we appreciate our aloneness, we can be ourselves and give ourselves most fully, and we no longer need others to save us or make us feel good about ourselves. Instead, we want to help them become *themselves* more fully as well. In this way, conscious love is born as a gift from our broken heart.

All the great spiritual traditions teach that single-minded pursuit of one's own happiness cannot lead to true satisfaction, for personal desires multiply endlessly, forever creating new dissatisfaction. Real happiness, which no one can ever take away, comes from breaking our heart open, feeling it radiating toward the world around us, and rejoicing in the well-being of others. Cherishing the growth of those we love exercises the larger capacities of our being and helps us ripen. Since their unfolding calls on us to develop all our finest qualities, we know that we are being fully used.

In an essay written in the 1920s, Orage maintained that conscious love was something extremely rare. Since people do not generally regard wisdom, truth, or creativity as central to an intimate relationship, he argued, they will seek out relationships based primarily on companionship or mutual self-interest. Yet though conscious love may still be rare today, it is no longer such a remote possibility. This is because unconscious love no longer works very well. As more and more couples discover that a relationship is most exciting when it helps them develop their deepest resources and finest qualities, conscious love may be seen as more of a necessity than a luxury. Thus all the current difficulties of relationships present us with a rare opportunity: to discover love as a sacred path, which calls on us to cultivate the fullness and depth of who we are.

THE FARTHER SHORE OF LOVE

In its final outreach, conscious love leads two lovers beyond themselves toward a greater connectedness with the whole of life. Indeed, two people's love will have no room to grow unless it develops this larger focus beyond themselves. The larger arc of a couple's love reaches out toward a feeling of kinship with all of life, what Teilhard de Chardin calls "a love of the universe." Only in this way can love, as he puts it, "develop in boundless light and power."

So the path of love expands in ever-widening circles. It begins at home—by first finding our seat, making friends with ourselves, and discovering the intrinsic richness of our being, underneath all our ego-centered confusion and delusion. As we come to appreciate this basic wholesomeness within us, we find that we have more to give to an intimate partner.

Further, as a man and a woman become devoted to the growth of awareness and spirit in each other, they will naturally want to share their love with others. The new qualities they give birth to—generosity, courage, compassion, wisdom—can extend beyond the circle of their own relationship. These qualities are a couple's "spiritual child"—what their coming together gives to the world. A couple will flourish when their vision and practice are not focused solely on each other, but also include this larger sense of community and what they can give to others.

From there, a couple's love can expand still further, as Teilhard suggests. The more deeply and passionately two people love each other, the more concern they will feel for the state of the world in which they live. They will feel their connection with the earth and a dedication to care for this world and all sentient beings who need their care. Radiating out to the whole of creation is the farthest reach of love and its fullest expression, which grounds and enriches the life of the couple. This is the great love and the great way, which leads to the heart of the universe.

Acknowledgments

WRITING THIS BOOK was a long, arduous journey in its own right, and I needed a great deal of help and support along the way. The people who read portions of the manuscript and gave me feedback during the ten years I worked on it are too numerous to mention here, but I want to express my thanks to all of them. Discussions with Ken Wilber, Robert Bly, Barbara Green, Joanne Martin Braun, Stephan Bodian, and Mary Goodell were particularly helpful at different points. I also want to acknowledge all the clients I have worked with over the years, whose willingness to explore the unknown in themselves provided me with a wealth of illustrative material for this book. (I have altered names and personal details about these individuals to protect privacy.)

Three people in particular deserve special recognition for the help they provided. Toinette Lippe offered encouragement over the course of many years, provided helpful feedback, and generously line-edited the manuscript on more than one occasion. Gregory Armstrong's editing and suggestions were also very helpful; he helped me rethink portions of the book and reshape several chapters. The greatest help of all came from my wife, Jennifer, who not only provided tremendous love and encouragement throughout the long process of completing the book, but also gave generously of her time in helping me wrestle the manuscript into final shape. She carefully edited it numerous times, helped me rewrite certain difficult passages, and added many helpful clarifications and elaborations of her own. To all these good friends, as well as to my teachers—especially Eugene Gendlin and Chögyam Trungpa—I am most grateful.

Further Resources

COUPLES IN THESE DIFFICULT TIMES need all the help they can get in finding their way. To develop greater awareness of what is happening in a relationship and free ourselves when we become bogged down, I particularly recommend mindfulness meditation and/or couple counseling.

MEDITATION

Centers where mindfulness meditation is taught and practiced can be found in most major urban centers throughout North America and Europe. In looking for such a center, be careful, for the word "meditation" is often used loosely to refer to a number of different activities, many of which have little to do with mindfulness or awareness. Mindfulness practices are taught within several different traditions, which may be listed in the telephone book under some of the following names: Insight Meditation, Vipassana, Zen, or Dharmadhatu. In addition, Shambhala Training, a meditation program based on the path of the warrior, has centers in many different areas. The national office, located at 2130 Arapahoe Ave., Boulder, CO 80302, (303) 444-7881, can give you the address of your nearest center.

COUNSELING

Couple counseling or therapy can often be quite helpful, even in a healthy, growing relationship. A disinterested third party can often help a couple find their way through tangles in which they become stuck. Sometimes a couple may need only one or two sessions with a skilled counselor to jog them loose from a harmful pattern; sometimes long-term work is useful in becoming aware of unconscious patterns and scripts that are operating. Unfortunately, many counselors and therapists are not well trained or highly skilled. The best way to find a skilled therapist is through a referral from a friend or acquaintance. Most importantly, if you go to see a professional, consult your own inner sense of whether this person is someone you trust and find helpful.

Notes

INTRODUCTION

1. Of course, there are many kinds of intimacy other than that between men and women—such as the parent–child relationship, deep friendship, and homosexual love—and no doubt many of the issues addressed in this book apply to them as well. However, I have chosen to limit my focus to the male–female connection because it is the area of greatest personal interest and concern to me.

CHAPTER 2

1. See E. T. Gendlin, *Focusing* (New York: Bantam, 1981).

CHAPTER 6

1. Any aspect of life can call forth this energized presence. For instance, the great modern saint, Mother Teresa, expresses unconditional passion in her work with poverty, disease, and death. The poor, the crippled, and the dying are doorways for her to the infinite.

2. The more people are cut off from their own being, the more they may go to extremes in order to connect with a source of "juice" in their life. The heroin addict needs his fix to feel alive, that is, unburdened by his loss of contact with his own being. Murderers are

often so dead inside that they try to feel alive by having power over life and death. Yet even in the worst addictions and debased activities, the same central motivation is present: the passionate desire to be fully connected with life. In this desire lies our basic human sanity and wholesomeness, even though what we do with it may lead to insanity and destruction.

3. In later centuries artists used romantic adoration in a similar way, as inspiration for their work. A classic example was Dante's love for Beatrice, a young girl he worshiped at a distance. His love for her inspired his art and provided him with spiritual vision. In Dante's *Divine Comedy,* Beatrice led him to the angelic realms of paradise.

4. Members of the Carmelite religious order practice what is called "bridal mysticism," becoming brides of Christ and using the energy of their "spiritual passion" to work their transformation. In the Hindu tradition, there is bhakti yoga, love and service to God. And in the Buddhist traditions of Tibet, devotion to the spiritual master plays an essential role on the path of enlightenment.

5. Perhaps only a small percentage of individuals who practiced courtly love were aware of the larger spiritual ramifications of what they were doing. Nonetheless, the overall thrust of that tradition was to use passionate devotion as a path of character development.

CHAPTER 9

1. The situation is very different in an extended family. If parents are physically absent or emotionally distant or disturbed, aunts, uncles, cousins, and grandparents are available to meet the growing child's needs for love and guidance. Traditional societies also had initiation rites at puberty to help the child separate from the parent of the opposite sex and identify with a larger community of elders of his or her own sex. The modern nuclear family has become a pressure cooker in which the parents' problems with love and intimacy are passed on directly to their children.

2. These two fears are interrelated at an emotional level. If our parents neglect or abandon us, we also feel engulfed by our intense feelings—of fear, need, and loss. Similarly, if a parent engulfs or dominates us, we also feel abandoned, for we do not feel seen or cared about for who we really are. Thus many people have both these sets of fears within them, and can play out either side of this dynamic with different partners.

3. I am choosing to focus on the abandonment/engulfment struggle here because it is one of the most destructive forms of polarization in relationships. Yet there are also many other ways in which couples may polarize. For example, one partner may be more disciplined and work-oriented, while the other is more carefree and playful. The harder he works, the more she wants to play. As they polarize, he becomes increasingly workaholic, while she may lose all sense of discipline, becoming increasingly unable to get anything done at all.

4. I am using the term *projection* here in a broader sense than the strict psychoanalytic meaning. Like a light that shines forth on the world around us, awareness usually passes through the "filmstrip" of our stories. As a result, we project these stories, along with all the preassigned roles they contain, onto the world and other people. What we generally see, then, is the movie we are projecting rather than things as they are in themselves. This is why many esoteric traditions say that life as we usually know it is a dream.

CHAPTER 12

1. This is not to say that women cannot also be pioneers or explorers. However, men more often feel something missing if they are not involved in exploring the edge of the unknown in some area of their lives. Women are more likely to feel unfulfilled if they are not involved in some form of relatedness or connectedness with people.

2. The posterior end of the corpus callosum, which is the fiber bundle carrying information between the two halves of the brain, is significantly larger and wider in women than in men. This finding provides a possible physiological basis for the widely observed fact that women are better at tasks requiring cooperation and communication between the two hemispheres of the brain, such as forming quick intuitive impressions of people based on verbal and visual cues simultaneously or having verbal access to the nonverbal world of their right hemisphere, while men are better at tasks that require separating the functions of the brain, such as talking or looking at a map while driving. See J. Smith & D. de Simone, *Sex and the Brain* (New York: Warner Books, 1983).

CHAPTER 13

1. The term *witch* has a number of different associations and meanings. The wicked witch of the fairy tales should be distinguished from the historical witch, who may have been a woman of genuine power in a culture that would not tolerate such power. Witches were most likely shamans who worked with herbs and earth energies for the purposes of healing and divination.

2. It was this kind of gentleness that Gandhi used to tame the British lion.

3. Of course, these principles also apply to the relations between yin and yang within each individual. Our yang strength can encourage and protect our yin tenderness. And our nourishing yin warmth can melt our rigid resistances and activate our yang urge to relate to life more expansively.

4. American men are in a state of deep crisis today. They are split between two conflicting identities: the rigid male, who wants to maintain domination and control, and the rebellious younger male, who finds nothing to emulate in older men and often winds up turning against male power altogether. Even our presidential politics of the past three decades reflect this split. On one side, Presidents Johnson, Nixon, and Reagan represent the rigid old man. On the other side, a Jimmy Carter or a Gary Hart insists on his right to remain a kid who is offended by having to grow up and assume genuine power and leadership. The only leader of the past three decades to bridge this gap and bring together the qualities of youthful exuberance and commanding presence—John Kennedy—was killed.

CHAPTER 14

1. A husband suffering from performance pressure feels obligated to be "turned on" even when he is not and to "provide" his wife with sexual fulfillment. Otherwise, he sees himself as a failure—as a man, as a husband, and perhaps as a human being as well. Perhaps he imagines that if he is armed with the latest know-how, he can overcome his anxiety about having to perform these feats. Yet his dependence on know-how only increases his alienation from his body, thus blocking him from the letting-go that is the source of sexual spontaneity.

Instead of living fully in his body, he tries to match his behavior to a mental picture. Sex becomes an act that he *performs,* under the direction and control of his thinking mind. This is a sure prescription for sexual dysfunction, as Masters and Johnson pointed out.

2. Indian Ayurvedic medicine pinpoints the *chakras* as the major psychophysical centers governing energy flow in the body, while Chinese medicine charts the acupuncture meridians. Both of these medical traditions grew out of systems of esoteric yoga. Although Western science and medicine do not recognize the subtle body, Eastern medicine sees its patterns of flow or blockage as the basis of the gross body's observable health or illness. The effect of the subtle body on the gross body is analogous to weather patterns: the storms and clearings we observe are the result of many forces in the cosmos that we do not directly observe. Therefore, Eastern medicine does not attack symptoms directly. Instead, it prefers to go "upstream" to address the underlying blockages and imbalances in a person's energy flow.

3. Some psychics and visionaries claim to see the subtle body as an aura of light or color.

4. We carry our overall response to a given individual inside us as a global "felt sense." A felt sense is what you will find if you turn inwardly and check out, for instance, what your father feels like to you, how he affects you, what the whole quality of your relationship with him is like. Your overall felt sense of your father has no definite form and may be hard to put into words, yet it has a distinctive "feel quality." The felt sense of your father will come into sharper focus if you compare it, for instance, with your felt sense of your mother, with whom you resonate in a very different way.

5. "He looked at her and inhaled her, she looked at him and inhaled him."—W. Somerset Maugham.

6. The subject of monogamy is a complex one that deserves a whole book in itself. There is only one way I can see monogamy working as an alive commitment, rather than as a form of deadening: through this kind of sacred awareness that allows two people to see each other as pure male and pure female, all men and all women.

CHAPTER 15

1. K. Dowman, *Sky Dancer* (London: Routledge & Kegan Paul, 1984).

2. I am borrowing this term from Riane Eisler's book, *The Chalice and the Blade* (San Francisco: Harper & Row, 1987).

Bibliography

To further explore the major themes and practices presented in this book, I particularly recommend the following:

Gendlin, E. *Focusing.* New York: Bantam, 1981.

A simple introduction to the Focusing method, which is an extremely helpful way of bringing awareness to unclear or difficult feelings, being present with them, and inquiring into them to discover new directions.

Hendrix, H. *Getting the Love You Want.* New York: Holt, 1988.

The best book I have seen on the material presented in Chapter 9 of this book. A thorough and helpful exploration of how our childhood wounds and scripts affect present relationships and how to work with the conflicts they raise.

Trungpa, C. *Shambhala: The Sacred Path of the Warrior.* Boston: Shambhala, 1984.

A powerful, inspiring, clear presentation of the path of the warrior, grounded in meditation practice.

Welwood, J. (Ed.). *Awakening the Heart: East/West Approaches to Psychotherapy and the Healing Relationship.* Boston: Shambhala, 1983.

Contains many helpful writings on working with our own states of mind and with those of others.

Welwood, J. (Ed.). *Challenge of the Heart: Love, Sex, and Intimacy in Changing Times.* Boston: Shambhala, 1985.

A companion volume to *Journey of the Heart.* Contains the most interesting, provocative, and helpful writings I came across while working on this book. Many of the writers mentioned in *Journey of the Heart* are represented here.

Wile, D. *After the Honeymoon: How Conflict Can Improve Your Relationship.* New York: Wiley, 1988.

The most useful practical book on couple communication I know.

Other recommended books containing material related to themes treated here:

De Rougemont, D. *Love in the Western World.* Translated by Montgomery Belgion. New York: Pantheon, 1956.

A classic work on passion and its development in Western culture. Even if you do not agree with de Rougemont's dour view of passion, his study is fascinating.

Evola, J. *The Metaphysics of Sex.* New York: Inner Traditions, 1983.

An interesting study of esoteric ideas and views of sexuality. Dense but illuminating.

Lawrence, D. H. *Phoenix: The Posthumous Papers of D. H. Lawrence.* Edited by Edward McDonald. London: Heinemann, 1936.

—————— *Phoenix II: Uncollected, Unpublished, and Other Prose Works by D. H. Lawrence.* Edited by Warren Roberts and Harry T. Moore. New York: Viking, 1970.

These two volumes contain Lawrence's best essays on love, sex, and marriage. Although Lawrence often can be annoyingly polemical, his essays contain some of the most passionate, eloquent, intelligent statements of the power of the man–woman connection to be found anywhere.

We have developed a training program based on the principles and practices in this book for individuals and couples who are interested in working with intimate relationship as path. These workshops, which include meditation practice and other experiential work, will be offered in various locations.

If you would like more information about these trainings, intensives for individual couples, or workshops for health professionals based on the principles in this book, please contact:

Journey of the Heart Seminars
P.O. Box 2173
Mill Valley, CA 94942
(415) 381-6077